CANCER

HANDBOOK

What's *Really* Working

Edited by

Lynne McTaggart

— like her work! Don't miss her Bk: The Field

Vital Health Publishing

Health ~ Nutrition

Bloomingdale, IL

The information contained in this book is not
intended to diagnose or prescribe for any medical condition. If you have a medical problem,
please consult with your primary care physician or holistic health care provider.

The Cancer Handbook: What's Really Working
Edited by Lynne McTaggart
2nd Edition U.S. Copyright ©2001, What Doctors Don't Tell You
Originally Published in the U.K. by What Doctor's Don't Tell
You, Copyright ©1997

Printed in the United States of America by United Graphics, Inc.,
Mattoon, IL on recycled paper using soy-based ink.

Published by:
    Vital Health Publishing
    P.O. Box 544
    Bloomingdale, IL 60108
    www.vitalhealth.net
    vitalhealth@compuserve.com
    (630) 876-0426

Cover photo inset: cancer cell microscopy image by Dr.
Kuruganti Murti.

ISBN: 1-890612-18-9

See Pg. 121 - TNF, Tumor Necrosis Factor
Pg 125 - Dr. Danopolous - 95% cure rate — Successful
Pg. 126 - Hydrogen Peroxide + Oxygen eyes
Tell mild ... eyes

For Edith Hubbard and

in memory of Olga McTaggart—

two courageous cancer patients

Pg 26 re psoriasis / ultra violet ray treatment

Pg 29 - cholesterol lowering drugs + Cancer

Pgs 45-46 + on: Mamography - is being
seen as of little use — is more
harmful than good - See
Pg 48 for bonus deal on pap smears.

Pg 114 - success shrinking tumors -
America shut down this.

Pg 116-117 - Polish Dr. - Dr. Burzynski's
struggle for FDA approval -
rotten Govt Control

Pg 118 Polish Dr. now ok'd to
operate clinic in Texas!

Contents

Introduction

The very word "cancer" fills us with dread, as though a death sentence had just been imposed. It is certainly one of the most feared of conditions—and increasingly one of the most widespread. At the start of this century, cancer claimed the life of one in 30; today it is estimated that it kills one in five. One in three of us in the West will have cancer at some point in our lives. It will also be the way most of us die.

However, little is really known about it. As there are many cancers, so there are many causes. We know that smoking is responsible for 90 percent of lung cancers in men and 77 percent in women, and that smokers are 30 percent more likely to develop cancer of the larynx.

All the billions of dollars of research we've thrown at cancer hasn't influenced survival one little bit. More people than ever are dying from the solid tumors that make up 90 percent of all cancers. You'd never know any of this if you talked to the average oncologist. Most would talk of the great strides made in chemotherapy, the new drugs, the new combinations of treatments. But the measure of how much this constitutes the treatment of desperation is in the language used—"rescue" therapies and "salvage" operations—and also the types of treatments being resorted to.

The medical spin-doctors have been particularly slick, instilling in the collective public mind a sense that we are winning the war. It's time to admit their deception. Take chemotherapy. No matter how many drugs or how high the dosage, it doesn't really work. Other treatments—the ones the American Cancer Society considers unproven—have better success rates. Once we all admit that, we can go forward.

And what about causes? Is there really such a thing as a cancer personality, someone more likely than others to develop the condition? Is it sparked by a poor diet? By power lines? By fluoridated water? By vegetable oils? By medicine itself? Very likely, there is a cumulative effect from all these things.

In this completely revamped and enlarged handbook, we look at some of these possible causes and how to avoid them. We also look at possible preventative actions, such as taking vitamins and other supplements. Should you already be a sufferer, or know someone who is, we examine the types of orthodox treatments on offer. We've devoted a large section of the handbook to alternative treatments. The most enigmatic feature of these treatments is that they might just work for you if you truly believe they will.

Of course, quack treatments that offer false hope should be stopped, but first we must establish that they are indeed quackery. What is fairly clear is that, when subjected to scientific scrutiny, most orthodox treatments do not work (chemotherapy, for instance, <u>has a success rate of just 5 percent</u>). Nonetheless, the cancer industry does not seem to run these treatments out of town for offering false hope. And, of course, with what we now understand about the influence of the mind on the body, if you truly believe that orthodox treatment will cure you, there's a reasonable likelihood that it could.

A booklet that covers so much ground would not have been possible without the help of many people. Our thanks are due to Dr. Ellen Grant, Fiona Bawdon, Simon Best, the Bristol Cancer Help Centre, Richard Walters, Deanne Pearson, Harald Gaier, and regular contributor Clive Couldwell for overseeing the editing. Finally, our special thanks go to Edith Hubbard, the mother of the publisher, to whom this book is dedicated. Her story is an inspiration to all those with cancer who have been condemned by the orthodoxy to die (see p. 159).

Lynne McTaggart

1

Possible causes

No easy answer

There is no one cause of cancer: cancer is not a dis-ease you can "catch", but rather a condition. Equally, there is probably no one trigger that can bring on the condition, but many factors—emotional, environ-mental, stress-related, dietary, medical—that can have a cumulative effect.

We all have cancer cells in our body; some immu-nologists reckon the body produces thousands every day. But as cancer pioneer Dr. Josef Issels pointed out, a healthy body cannot develop cancer because it has a defense system that can recognize cancer cells and reject them. Cancer can, therefore, only develop in an unhealthy body or one whose immune system is not functioning properly.

Research carried out by American psychologist Lawrence LeShan in the 1970's indicated that there can be a cancer personality—someone who because of their life and emotional responses is more likely to develop cancer. For instance, the cancer patients he interviewed tended to have a difficult childhood, an early sense of inadequacy, unsatisfactory parental relationships, an inability to vent their emotions and a defeatist attitude.

But, then, not everyone with that profile will go on to develop cancer, just as not every smoker gets lung cancer. Here, then, are some likely causes, or factors that just may tip the balance. One possible cause could be the lack of vitamins and minerals that would be supplied by a healthy diet. The causes we have examined in this section are not so much a lack of something, but an overexposure to hazards.

FAMILY HISTORY

Interestingly, family history, often fingered by medicine as a likely suspect—seems not to play the vital role we've all been led to believe. For instance, the link between a family history of breast cancer and a woman's likelihood of developing the disease is smaller than suggested earlier, according to American research.

Earlier studies have suggested that there is a strong correlation—which has been enough to prompt some doctors to suggest that women in supposedly high-risk groups should have "prophylactic mastectomies"—that is, just-in-case surgery to remove their healthy breasts—to avoid developing the disease. However, a study of 117,988 women aged 30 to 55 found that the "risk associated with a mother or sister history of breast cancer is smaller than suggested by earlier retrospective studies. Overall, within this population of middle-aged women, only 2.5 percent of breast cancer cases are attributable to a positive family history."

They suggest that the size of the increased risk identified in earlier studies may in part be explained by "heightened awareness or over-reporting of family history by patients with breast cancer, whereas control patients may be less aware of all breast cancer diagnoses in their family" (*JAMA,* July 21, 1993).

CONTRACEPTIVES
The Pill

In the 30 years since the advent of the Pill, evidence has mounted indicating a relationship between it and breast and cervical cancer. The cervical cancer link is taken as read, but is considered an acceptable risk because cervical smear tests will catch it in time.

Dr. Ellen Grant has been pointing out the dangers of the Pill for many years. In her book, *The Bitter Pill* (Elm Tree Books, 1985), Dr. Grant describes it as "the most powerful immunosuppressant known in medicine." By far the commonest type of cancer in young women which can be caused by the Pill is cervical, she points out. Even when the Pill was first introduced into Britain in 1961, scientists already knew that estrogens caused cancer in animals. However, animal studies supposedly demonstrated that use of a combined pill containing progestogen, an artificial progesterone, could protect against this cancer developing.

In 1968, according to a report in "World Medicine", two American studies had recorded a higher incidence of early cervical cancer, which is known as "carcinoma in situ." One unpublished study, by a Professor Weid of America, estimated that the risk was increased six times from three in 1000 to 18 in 1000 for those who had taken the Pill for five years or more, although among 40,000 women screened, only 500 were still using the Pill after five years.

Officially, registration for cervical carcinoma in situ began in 1965. At that time a young woman aged 15 to 24 had a less than one in 100,000 chance of developing a positive smear. By 1978 the figures for England and Wales had increased tenfold from 0.8 per 100,000 to 8.5 per 100,000 and had increased by 1220 percent by 1981.

In 1972 very few single women in the country had ever used the Pill (9 percent), but by 1982 young unmarried women made up the majority of first-time

Pill users at most clinics. The largest family planning clinic in Europe—the Margaret Pyke Centre in London—reported in The Lancet that one in 25 women attending had a positive smear and that there had been a sharp increase in serious abnormalities.

A large-scale American study of Pill users in Walnut Creek, California, had 37 cases of cervical cancer among Pill users under 40 and one case in the control group. Again, although smokers were statistically more likely to be affected than non-smokers, the actual figures were nearly the same—14 smokers and 18 non-smokers. What this means is that cancer is more prevalent among non-smoking Pill users than among smokers who don't take the Pill.

Dr. Albert Singer said at a meeting of the Women's National Cancer Control Campaign in London in June 1985 that a new incurable type of cervical cancer was becoming epidemic. The three-year survival rate for women under 24 had declined from 93 percent to only 72 percent between 1977 and 1979. Half the under 40s inflicted with invasive cervical cancer now die within five years or less. When human papilloma virus type 16 (genital warts) was present in the male partner, 80 percent of the women developed pre-cancerous smears. A 1985 World Health Organization study from eight developing countries showed invasive cancer increased with length of Pill use.

But it is not the only cancer linked to the Pill. Professor Malcolm Pike and his team from California presented their data in The Lancet in October 1983, showing that breast cancer was increased four- or five-fold among women who had taken the Pill for six years or more before they were 25, and the risk was greater for high-dose progestogen pills. It was the third study to find that young women who had begun the Pill before they were 25, or before their first full-term pregnancy, had an increased risk of breast cancer and the risk went up the longer the Pill had been taken.

The latest damning news comes from a study by the Department of Epidemiology at the Netherlands Cancer Institute.

In the Dutch study, 97 percent of the 918 Dutch women with invasive breast cancer, diagnosed before age 36, had taken the Pill. For those starting before age 20 the increase was 3.5 times risk. Longer use increased the risk, with trends increasing sharply for younger and older takers.

Their largest group of cases in this study were aged 36-45, had taken the Pill for less than four years and had a 1.4 increased risk.

Klim McPherson, an epidemiologist at the London school of Tropical Medicine, has estimated that because of the latent period, this risk could increase to one in four among early age longer-term Pill takers. The risk is increased by 30 times if a near relation has the disease due to breast cancer genes. Any menopausal estrogens further ups their risk 3.5 times.

Depo-Provera

The injectable long-lasting contraceptive, Depo-Provera, doubles the risk of breast cancer among women who have taken it for less than five years. It seems to be at its most dangerous in the first few years of use.

This startling discovery was made soon after the hormone was finally approved for marketing in the United States. Many countries had held back from granting a license because of the breast cancer risks associated with the progesterone contraceptive. The sudden change of heart by the American Food and Drug Administration (FDA) was caused by two studies, from New Zealand and by the World Health Organization, which both concluded that the contraceptive did not heighten the cancer risk.

However, a closer analysis of the data shows that the risk in fact doubles in the first five years of taking the hormone, and then drops to almost nothing after that. Researchers believe that Depo-Provera might quicken tumor promotion and growth. If it

does, its potency must be far stronger than doctors
believe because just one injection seems able to
influence cancer growth for the next five years
(*JAMA*, March 8, 1995).

Condoms

Having been lauded as the safest contraceptive, the
male condom is now thought to cause cancer in the
woman, and may also make her infertile.

Rather than the condom itself, the culprit appears
to be talc, a dry lubricant on the surface of condoms.
Studies have shown talc to cause ovarian cancer as
well as fibrosis on fallopian tubes, causing infertility.
Strangely, the American FDA recognized the dangers of talc on surgical gloves, and banned the
process, but allowed its continued application on
condoms.

Writing in *JAMA*, Candace Kasper and P J
Chandler of Dallas, Texas fear there could be a major
outbreak of ovarian cancer in years ahead. They also
urge condom manufacturers to stop applying talc
(*JAMA*, March 15, 1995).

OTHER TREATMENTS

In-vitro fertilization (IVF)

The dangers inherent in the Pill and Depo-Provera
seem to hold good for other interventions which

also muck about with the body's natural hormonal balance.

Doctors are beginning to fear that assisted-conception techniques such as IVF could be causing cancers, especially ovarian cancer.

The long-term effects of the treatment are not known, simply because nobody has bothered to research them. Incomplete studies have pointed to a rise in endometrial cancer, breast cancer and ovarian cancer, but the findings are not conclusive.

When the Australian National Health and Medical Research Council looked for reactions to the drugs used in the procedure, they found just 37 reports filed with the authorities since 1971, which demonstrated the bias of voluntary drug surveillance programs, they concluded.

Hormone Replacement Therapy (HRT)

HRT is another hormonal treatment which older women—who may already have been on the Pill in their younger years—are increasingly being encouraged to take. This drug can increase your breast cancer risk by 60 percent, according to three large-scale reviews of many of the large studies to date.

It is acknowledged that when a woman with a womb takes estrogen on its own, she increases her chances up to 20-fold of getting endometrial cancer after several years. This is because estrogen causes rapid proliferation of endometrial cells (as it does in pregnancy). This risk can continue for up to five years after stopping HRT.

To counteract this, most women are given the additional artificial hormone progestogen (progestin in the US) for 10-12 days per month, which imitates the second half of the menstrual cycle, producing withdrawal bleeding. Researchers from the Menopause Clinic at King's College School of Medicine and Dentistry found that endometrial stimulation in women given HRT implants occurred for an average of two years after the treatment was finished (*BMJ*, February 17, 1990). What this means is, to lower your risk of getting endometrial cancer, you would have to take oral progestogen for two years or more after the estrogen in the implant has been exhausted.

Long-term use of HRT and the Pill also greatly increases the risk of breast cancer in older women, researchers have found.

During a study of the bone mineral density of 6854 women aged over 65, researchers found that women with increased bone mineral density have a far higher chance of developing breast cancer. As bone mineral density is increased by long-term usage of estrogen and progestogens, such as in HRT and the contraceptive pill, it follows that the primary indicator for breast cancer risk is hormone supplementation, and not bone mineral density, as the researchers have suggested. Insulin levels can also affect the level of bone density so that, too, should be included in the equation.

The researchers, from the University of Pittsburgh, say their findings mean that people should think more carefully about taking HRT for anything other than osteoporosis (*JAMA*, 1996; 276: 1404-08)—although that supposed benefit of the drug, too, has been discredited (see WDDTY *Guide to The Menopause*).

HRT may also increase the risk of death in countries where there is a low level of heart disease. Researchers there found that, rather than protecting women from fatal heart problems, HRT was increasing the risks in Italian women. The chances of developing breast cancer increased by up to 1.46 times if the therapy was used for between 15 and 20 years, while the risks for heart disease increased by 0.88 times after five years (*BMJ*, 1996; 313: 687).

Diethylstilbestrol (DES)

DES is another fertility-type treatment linked with cancer. Women who took this miscarriage prevention drug during pregnancy in the Fifties and Sixties have a "statistically significant" increased risk of developing breast cancer (*JAMA*, April 28, 1993).

Researchers at the Boston University School of Public Health studied a group of 3029 women who had taken DES and the same number who had not been exposed to the drug. They found 325 cases of breast cancer within the groups, 185 among the DES women and 140 among the unexposed women.

"The incidence rate of breast cancer per 100,000 woman-years was 172.3 among exposed women and 134.1 among the unexposed," they concluded. When other factors, such as age and age when pregnant were taken into account, the relative risk associated with DES exposure was 1.35 times that of those not exposed to the drug. The study did not bear out earlier findings which suggested the risk increases over time.

The children of these women may also face a far greater risk of developing breast cancer. Specialists from the British Columbia Cancer Agency have reported two cases—both daughters of DES patients, aged 28 and 34—who have breast cancer.

DES was used extensively to treat possible miscarriage and infertility up until 1971 in the US, and until 1978 in Europe, when the drug was removed from the market. DES is one of the few external factors accepted as increasing the risk of breast cancer among women; the other two are alcohol and ionizing radiation. The risk among DES mothers increases by 35 percent.

It has been recognized that DES daughters are more likely to develop cervical cancer, and suffer premature births and miscarriages, but it was thought the breast cancer risks were not passed on: "We may now begin to see the full extent of its effects as DES daughters grow older," say the doctors in a letter to The Lancet (1996; 348: 331).

Growth hormones

It is not just women who are at risk because of medicine's hormonal meddling. Men may be more likely to develop prostate cancer if their mothers took pregnancy and growth hormones when they were in the womb.

This link has been made by Swedish researchers after they studied the birth records of 250 men who developed prostate cancer, and compared them with records of 691 others, 80 of whom died from prostate cancer. They found that those born full-term, and with a high birth weight and height, were more likely to develop the cancer. Conversely, those whose mothers had pre-eclampsia, or who themselves were born prematurely, were much less likely to develop prostate cancer.

Although there was no direct proof that the mothers were taking hormones, the scientists believe the data support earlier hypotheses of a link between hormones and prostate cancer (*BMJ*, 1996; 313: 337-340—See also WDDTY's *Guide to Men's Health* for more information on prostate cancer).

X-rays

As many as 250 cases of fatal cancer each year are caused by unnecessary x-rays, according to the Royal College of Radiologists and the National Radiological Protection Board. The two bodies produced a set of guidelines to cut radiation exposure by half without affecting the quality of care. The report estimated that at least one-fifth of all x-rays were unnecessary and that routine chest x-rays, x-rays to diagnose lower back pain and mammograms for low-risk women under 50 were all unnecessary.

Dental x-rays may be particularly dangerous as they are often taken by untrained staff.

At least one leading expert blames the high rate of breast cancer in the US on the liberal use of medical x-rays. Many women were given high doses of x-rays by doctors before the carcinogenic effects of radiation were appreciated. Probably 75 percent of all the 182,000 cases of breast cancer reported in the US every year are due to medical x-rays, he says.

The claims are made by John Gofman, Professor of Molecular and Cell Biology at the University of California, after he studied medical research going as far back as 1910. But Gofman's conclusion has not impressed many cancer experts who fear that women may be deterred from having mammograms, which supposedly detect early cancers.

Since preparing his book, *Preventing Breast Cancer*, Gofman has increased his estimates of cancers caused by x-rays to 90 percent. He points out that x-ray therapy was once very prevalent, used to to treat a range of conditions from pneumonia to acne and hair removal. Gofman estimates that women's breasts receive 0.4 rad of medical x-rays a year for each year of life; comparing that dosage with the levels suffered by Japanese atomic bomb survivors, he reckoned that 114,000 women, or 62 percent of those diagnosed every year with breast cancer, could blame x-rays as the cause. A more realistic figure would be 75 percent, he concluded (*Preventing Breast Cancer*, by Dr. John Gofman, Committee for Nuclear Responsibility, San Francisco, California).

However, a recent study rejects Gofman's findings. The US National Cancer Institute has assessed the breast cancer risk among radiologic technicians, and found that their work was not a contributory factor (*JAMA*, August 2, 1995).

Meanwhile, according to the National Radiological Protection Board and the Royal College of Radiologists in the UK, unnecessary radiation from x-rays may be responsible for between 100 and 250 of the 160,000 cancer deaths in the UK every year and perhaps 1000 cancer deaths a year in the US.

In the US, a study by the National Cancer Institute (*JAMA*, March 13, 1991) found a link between x-rays and multiple myeloma—a form of bone cancer. They looked at more than 25,000 x-rays and concluded that with myeloma sufferers "there was consistent evidence for a dose-response trend regardless of the lagging interval. The most frequently exposed were at highest risk, reaching four-fold."

In 1991, the National Academy of Sciences reported that estimates of lifetime cancer risk following relatively low doses of radiation may be as much as four times larger than previously thought (NAS—National Research Council. *Health Effects of Exposure to Low Levels of Ionizing Radiation*. Washington DC: National Academy Press).

All radiation is harmful (and your body never "forgets" the radiation it has received), but some groups are particularly at risk. Unborn children are especially susceptible and pregnant women should avoid all x-rays except in extreme, life-threatening situations.

The link between exposure of fetuses to radiation and childhood cancer is well documented (*Int. J. Cancer*, 1990; 46: 362-365; *British J. of Cancer*, 1990; 62: 152-68). In *Health Shock* (Prentice-Hall, 1982), M. Weitz claims that the x-rays given to about a quarter of all pregnant women during the 1950's and 1960's "caused between 5 and 10 percent of all childhood cancers in America and Western Europe."

Once they are born, children remain at increased risk. In *Medicine on Trial* (Pantheon), John Gofman and Egan O'Connor claim that "a newly-born child is about 300 times more sensitive than a 55-year-old to induction of cancer by radiation." Five-year-old children are "about five times more likely to get later radiation-induced cancer than an adult given the same radiation dose at age 35," they add.

THE ENVIRONMENT
Fluoridated water
An American government study has confirmed that fluoride added to water causes cancer in laboratory animals. The study, conducted by the National Toxicology Program and overseen by the American Public Health Service, looked at the link between water fluoridation and mouth, liver and bone cancers in rats and mice.

The results, interpreted by John Yiamouyiannis,

President of the Safe Water Foundation in Ohio (writing in the *Townsend Letter for Doctors,* an American journal) showed, among the rats exposed to the fluoridated water:

- pre-cancerous changes in cells in the mouth;
- an increase in the incidence of tumors and cancers in the mouth;
- a rare form of bone cancer;
- an increase in the tumors in the thyroid.

The mice exposed to fluoridated water had a rare form of liver cancer. "The types of cancer caused by fluoride in rats and mice may be entirely different than the types of cancer caused by that same substance in humans," wrote Yiamouyiannis, who has performed epidemiological studies on the effects of fluoride.

The animals were given higher doses of fluoride than humans would be exposed to, in order to adjust for the short time of their exposure to fluoride. Also, according to the study, says Yiamouyiannis "man is generally more vulnerable" than the experimental animals to the carcinogenic effects. Nevertheless, the doses of fluoride linked to a higher cancer risk were between 1/10 to 1/50 of that of benzene, another established carcinogen.

Pesticides

Pesticides like DDT may also trigger breast cancer. Several recent studies have shown a fourfold increase in the risk of developing breast cancer among women with high bodily levels of DDT. The US has controlled the use of DDT to levels 5000 percent below that of other developed countries, although environmentalists fear these controls could be relaxed with the General Agreement on Tariffs and Trade (*JAMA*, April 20, 1994).

Power lines

Living near power lines may also put you at greater risk. Evidence shows that the relatively low levels of electromagnetic fields (EMFs) from main electricity or power lines can raise the chances of your child getting leukemia by three or four times.

In 1979, two American researchers, Nancy Wertheimer and Ed Leeper, published the first major Western study linking EMFs from power lines and domestic wiring configurations to an increase in childhood cancer (*Am. J. Epidemiol*, 1979; 109: 273-84).

There are some 12 studies of residential exposure to EMFs in Britain, of which nine show an elevated risk of childhood cancer; the three studies which do not have been criticized for their methodology. The density of magnetic fields are measured in what are called teslas. On average, the positive studies have found a significantly increased risk at 200-300 nanotesla—a nanotesla (nT) is one thousandth of a millionth tesla. However, the National Radiological Protection Board (NRPB) will only begin to investigate at a level of 1600 microtesla (uT)—a millionth of a tesla—a difference of between 5400- and 8000-fold.

An average household level is 70 nT; the level beneath power lines can rise to over 1000 nT.

In the US the situation is very different. Many researchers advocate a general policy of "prudent avoidance"—recommending a number of safety measures to avoid excessive exposure. At least 10 states have restrictions on the level of EMFs allowed in houses built near power lines.

Electric and magnetic fields surround all electrical conductors, including power lines, appliances and the wiring in your house. EMFs are comprised of electrical fields and magnetic fields. Electrical fields can be shielded by walls and trees and, unless you live near a power line, aren't a problem. Magnetic fields, on the other hand, are generated by electrical current whenever you use electricity. They can travel through walls and only be shielded against with lead shields, and careful design of wiring and electrical equipment.

Drs Maria Feychting and Anders Ahlbom, at

the Institute of Environmental Medicine at the Karolinska Institute in Stockholm, conducted a large-scale epidemiological study, which found that children exposed to average domestic EMFs of 300 nT or more had almost four times the rate of leukemia than expected (*American Journal of Epidemiology*, 1993; 138: 467-81).

The subjects were the 500,000 who had all lived within 300 meters of the country's network of 220 and 400 kV powerlines between 1960 and 1985, of whom 142 children developed cancer.

The study established for the first time a clear dose-response correlation between levels of magnetic field exposure and increased incidence of leukemia. Children exposed to more than 100 nT EMFs had twice the incidence of leukemia than those exposed to less than 100 nT, those exposed to above 200 nT nearly three times, and those exposed to over 300 nT nearly four times. Similar results were obtained when exposure was defined by proximity to power lines.

Such was the impact of this and another study released at the same time, which also found a strong link with brain tumors in men occupationally exposed to EMFs (Cancer Causes Control, 1993; 4: 465-76), that Sweden's National Board for Industry and Technology (NUTEK) formally announced that it "would act on the assumption that there is a connection between exposure to power frequency magnetic fields and cancer, in particular, childhood cancer."

In addition, NUTEK has advocated a moratorium on erecting power lines creating fields of 200 nT near houses and school buildings until further guidance has been drafted.

The first link between female breast cancer and exposure to electromagnetic fields began with studies of the rare cases of breast cancer in men. In 1989, Dr. Genevieve Matanoski and her colleagues at the John Hopkins School of Public Health in Baltimore, Maryland, found that there was significantly more than expected cases of breast cancer among New York State central telephone technicians (*The Lancet*, March 23, 1990).

This was followed by studies showing that telephone linesmen, electricians and electric power workers all suffer an increased breast cancer risk (*Am. J. Epidm.*, 1991; 134: 340-7; *The Lancet*, 1990; 336: 1596 and 1992; 339: 1482-3).

In 1992, the first connection was made between EMF exposure and female breast cancer. Dr. Dana Loomis of the University of North Carolina observed a 40 percent increased mortality from the disease in female electrical workers, twice the number of deaths expected in women between 45 and 54 (*J.*

Nat. Cancer Inst., 1994; 86: 921-5).

But the study that has prompted most interest is the recent work by Loscher in Germany, which has now confirmed a relationship between levels of magnetic fields and likelihood of developing breast cancer in rats treated with a chemical carcinogen (*Carcinogenesis,* 1995; 16: 1199-25). The higher the magnetic field, the more likely the rats were to get cancer.

One clue as to the precise mechanism by which EMFs can trigger cancer came from Loscher's rats. When exposed to 10,000 nT, the rats' night time blood melatonin levels decreased by one-third. Melatonin, produced by the pineal gland, the body's master control gland, is a powerful antioxidant that scavenges excessive free radicals in the body. If allowed to build up in the body, free radicals can damage DNA and increase cancer risk, as well as human degenerative disorders like heart, Alzheimer's and Parkinson's diseases.

We're now learning that melatonin is extremely sensitive to magnetic fields. A growing number of researchers, led by Dr. Russel Reiter at the University of Texas Health Science Center in San Antonio, believe that the suppression of melatonin production is the most likely link between EMFs and all cancer (*J. Pineal Research,* 1995; 18: 1-11). At the 1994 annual meeting of the Bioelectromagnetics

Society, Robert Liburdy, at the University of California's Lawrence Berkeley Laboratories, reported that he had observed that magnetic fields of between 600 nT and 1,200 nT, exposed to cultured human breast cancer cells, suppressed the anti-cancer action of melatonin, allowing cancer cells to multiply (*J. Pineal Research,* 1993; 14: 89-97).

A leaked draft report on EMF exposure guidelines for extremely low frequency electric and magnetic fields by the US National Council on Radiation Protection tacitly acknowledged the danger: "Disturbance of the normal diurnal melatonin rhythm is associated with altered estrogen receptor formation in the breast, a line of experimental evidence now under study for possible links between ELF field exposure and human breast cancer."

EMFs

In the light of mounting evidence, everyone, but particularly women, should reduce their exposure to EMFs, both at work and in the home.

Sit at least four feet from the sides and rear of VDUs (where the highest fields are emitted). In the home, the major source of elevated fields of exposure is usually the bedroom. If you already have breast cancer, you might be well advised to check the levels of magnetic field in your bedroom overnight.

Household power linked to cancer

As well as there being dangers from from external sources, ordinary household electrical gadgets—vacuum cleaners, ovens and food mixers—can also cause cancer.

A leaked report, prepared for the US Government's radiation advisers, recommends safety limits for exposure to electromagnetic fields that are 5,000 times lower than international safety levels, and 8,000 lower than current British ones.

The National Council on Radiation Protection says that EMF exposure should never be higher than 0.2 uT. If introduced, most household gadgets would be considered unsafe; vacuum cleaners and drills, for example, have a range of between 2 and 20 uT, food mixers between 0.6 and 10, hair dryers between 0.01 and 7, dishwashers between 0.6 and 3, washing machines between 0.15 and 3, and electric ovens between 0.15 and 0.5.

When these appliances are switched off general household levels of EMF are considered safe, unless the home is within 25 meters or less of a power line. If a 400kV line is 25 meters from the home, this will increase general EMF levels to 8 uT.

The report, prepared by an 11-man committee over nine years, also points to research showing that exposure to even weak EMFs can affect the production of melatonin, and makes the possible link with breast cancer.

Ultraviolet A radiation (PUVA)

Long-term exposure to ultraviolet A radiation has been shown to cause skin cancer. Psoriasis sufferers treated with ultraviolet A radiation therapy may simply be swapping one skin condition for another far more serious. If they have had more than 250 treatments, their risks of developing skin cancer increase nearly nine times. The risks worsen with the length and frequency of treatment.

Patients seem to be at no more risk than the general population from developing malignant melanoma during the first 15 years of treatment. After that, however, the risks rise alarmingly to 5.4 times during the following five years and to 8.9 times if the patient has had more than 250 exposures to PUVA.

Researchers from Harvard Medical School tracked 1380 psoriasis patients who were first treated with the ultraviolet A radiation therapy PUVA in either 1975 or 1976.

PUVA—psoralen plus ultraviolet A radiation—has become a mainstay treatment for severe psoriasis since its introduction in the mid-1970s. Although it was known to cause skin cancer, it was always associated with skin type, the cumulative load of ultraviolet A radiation and earlier cancer-causing treatments. The Harvard study is the first to observe that the risk worsens over time.

In an accompanying editorial, Klaus Wolff from the University of Vienna said that medicine needs to decide whether PUVA treatment should be stopped "since the death of a single patient with melanoma outweighs any other benefits that may be derived from such treatment." Dr. Wolff concluded that the treatment should continue, although patients given long-term PUVA therapy need to be carefully observed throughout their lives (*New Eng. J. Med.,* 1997; 336: 1041-5).

Sunbathing

Is skin cancer caused by too much sunbathing? This much-cherished view has been challenged by researchers from Yale. They found a link between sunburn and a melanoma that may form later at the exact same spot, but not with the position of any tumor. They were unable to explain why quite a number of melanomas form on parts of the body that are rarely, if ever, exposed to the sun (*Int. Jrnl. of Cancer,* 1996; 67: 636-46).

Much of what we're told about the dangers of sunbathing is wrong. Sunscreens may in fact increase the risk, while advice on keeping out of the sun seems to be too simplistic.

Studies show that there is a melanoma epidemic going on; in New South Wales, Australia, for example, cases have doubled in the past two years, while other surveys have shown a rise of up to 43 percent a year. And all this at a time when public awareness of melanoma, and ways to supposedly prevent it, couldn't be higher.

The fact is that the medical profession knows very little about melanoma, but what it does know does not bear out the advice generally handed out. For example, scientists know that people who are constantly out in the sun are less likely to develop melanoma than those who go out in it only intermittently, and there seems an important interaction between skin type and the disease.

Scientists don't know which part of the sun's rays is responsible for bringing on the disease, or the role and importance of ultraviolet radiation in tumor growth. Without this knowledge, sunscreens are useless, and actually may be responsible for bringing on the cancer in some cases.

One researcher who has studied the latest epidemic in New South Wales is suggesting that there could be two types of melanoma: one which is responsible for the thin lesions which can be easily removed, and a second form which generates thicker lesions, and which may be pre-existing. In other words, they were there irrespective of sun exposure. If his supposition is accurate, it would only mean that melanoma follows the pattern of other, better-understood, cancers where most skin cancer cells prove to be harmless, and may even regress (*BMJ*, January 20, 1996).

DRUGS

Besides environmental causes, many medical treatments are being implicated as contributing to the cancer statistics. The latest evidence points to a number of drugs, which appear to be carcinogenic.

Cholesterol drugs

Cholesterol-lowering drugs may cause cancer, a possibility that doctors and regulators would have been aware of had they read the research properly.

Scientists from the University of California have re-analyzed the data published in *The Physicians' Desk Reference* the American drug reference bible, to discover a definite link between most of the popular cholesterol-lowering drugs and cancer. Tests carried out on rodents show the carcinogenic effects of the drugs, especially if taken longer-term.

Their findings cast a shadow over the millions of

users of the drugs around the world. They are some of the most popularly prescribed drugs; their usage has increased 10-fold in the past decade and, in 1992 in the US alone, 26 million prescriptions for the drugs were written out.

The Californian researchers, Dr. Thomas Newman and Stephen Hulley, fear that modern medicine may be preparing a massive cancer time bomb, its effects not fully realized for another 30 years. Despite this, the researchers conclude that the benefits of the drugs outweigh the risks among those with high blood cholesterol, especially men—provided they have taken the drug for under five years. Those not at high risk from raised cholesterol levels should avoid the treatment, the researchers advise, particularly if they have a life expectancy greater than 20 years.

But if all these risks were already in the data submitted to the Food and Drug Administration, how did the drugs get approved in the first place? The Californian researchers note that the drugs were approved on the basis of less than 10 years' clinical trials, yet the full effects of the drugs may not become clear for 30 years.

The carcinogenic effects of two of the drugs, lovastatin and gemfibrozil, were discussed in a drug advisory committee meeting. The drug manufacturer representative of lovastatin "downplayed the importance of the studies," the researchers say. The data were also prepared in milligrams per kilogram of body weight, which may have confused the committee.

After these revelations, the committee recommended that gemfibrozil should be used only as a drug of last resort, after exercise, diet and weight loss had failed to bring down cholesterol levels. The popularity of the drug since then suggests it has been far more widely used than the committee wanted (*JAMA*, January 3, 1996).

Fertility drugs

Fertility drugs are some of the latest medications to be associated with cancer, specifically of the ovary and breast.

In the US at least 12.5 million courses of fertility drugs have been prescribed since they were launched in the 1960s. In January 1993, the US FDA asked drug manufacturers to add the risk of ovarian cancer to the possible adverse reactions listed on fertility drug labels such as clomiphene citrate (Clomid) and menotrophins. The decision was prompted by an evaluation of the results of 12 studies (analyzed by the American Collaborative Ovarian Cancer Group based at Stanford University, California, and published in the *American Journal of Epidemiology*) on risk factors for ovarian cancer. These found that the risk of invasive ovarian cancer among infertile women who had taken fertility drugs was almost three times that of fertile women, and that infertile women who had not taken fertility drugs were not at increased risk (*Lancet*, 1993; 341: 234).

The link between fertility drugs and ovarian cancer is in keeping with the two main theories regarding the possible causes of ovarian cancer. The first is that the surface of the ovaries are damaged each time a woman ovulates and that this may eventually trigger the cancer. Therefore by increasing ovulation, fertility drugs are increasing a woman's risk of developing cancer. The American study also revealed that women who ovulate less often—through having a number of pregnancies and breastfeeding their children, or by taking the contraceptive pill which prevents ovulation, for example—are at less risk of ovarian cancer. The second theory is that exposure to high levels of pituitary gonadtropins (which clomiphene stimulates the release of) increases the risk of ovarian cancer.

Ovarian cancer is the fifth most common cancer in women, and because it is not usually discovered until it is in an advanced state, most women die from it. It is also most common in women over 50, and three times more common in women who have never had children. So we may only just be starting to see ovarian cancers caused by fertility drugs taken by women in the 1960s. As more and more women receive treatment for infertility there may be an increasing number of cases of ovarian cancer over the ensuing decades.

One study found that women taking clomiphene ran an increased risk of ovarian tumors whether or not they had ovarian abnormalities. They discovered 11 invasive or borderline malignant ovarian tumors compared with an expected 4.4. Nine of the women had taken clomiphene. Their results also indicated that the risk of a tumor is dependent on the length of time a woman takes the drug. Those who had taken clomiphene for less than 12 menstrual cycles were at no increased risk, whereas those who had used it for 12 or more cycles were at considerably increased risk, according to the researchers.

However, the study found no increase in the risk of ovarian tumors associated with the use of human chorionic gonadotropin, which stimulates the ovaries to produce estrogen and progesterone, although it may also induce ovulation. Although the findings suggested that prolonged use of clomiphene increased the risk of ovarian tumors, larger studies are needed to test the hypothesis (*N. Engl. J. Med*, Sept 22, 1994; 331: 771-6.)

The French are currently conducting a large-scale epidemiological study to determine the risk of ovarian cancer in women who have been treated with ovulation-inducing drugs. There are about 3200 deaths from ovarian cancer every year in France and about 4000 new cases (*Lancet*, Oct 22, 1994).

Blood pressure drugs

New research suggests that calcium antagonists, given to treat hypertension (high blood pressure), cause cancer. They have already been blamed for increasing heart attack risk and causing stomach bleeding.

The new finding was made by researchers in the US and Italy, who tracked 750 elderly patients treated for hypertension for four years. Those who were taking calcium antagonists suffered a rate of cancer double that for the other groups, who were prescribed ACE inhibitors or beta blockers (*The Lancet*, 1996; 348: 49).

Several classes of drugs—including diuretics and antihypertensives (for lowering of blood pressure)—are suspected as being possible causes of cancer of the kidney. A new study has re-examined a number of possible causes, and included information from seven studies that linked various cancers to high blood pressure.

The possible link between hypertension and cancer

was first noted in 1975, but it has never been confirmed. Diuretics were suspected as being a cause of renal (kidney) cancer in 1992, but larger trials have not confirmed this.

Another suspect has been the beta blocker atenolol, when it was noted that cancer was twice as common in hypertensive sufferers taking the therapy. Antihypertensive drugs have also been pinpointed as a possible cause of renal cancer in several studies (*Hypertension*, 1996; 28: 321-4).

SURGERY

Breast surgery

Although surgery for cancer is touted as being the first port of call in cancer treatment (see p 107), it also appears to increase the risks of the disease spreading. Surgery for breast cancer also increases the risk of relapse or death within three years following the procedure, according to UK cancer specialist Michael Baum.

Mr Baum, based at the Royal Marsden Hospital in London, said that women who have surgery for breast cancer are not necessarily in the clear if they survive the initial three years. Relapse or death can reoccur years later, although it is a less dramatic peak the second time, he said. This goes against current thinking, which suggests that the disease continues to develop at a constant rate (*The Lancet,* January 27, 1996).

Vasectomies

Whether it's artificial hormones to stop women becoming pregnant, or vasectomies for men, tinkering with the body's reproductive ability seems to increase cancer risk. Men who have had vasectomies are more likely to develop prostate cancer, according to two US studies of more than 73,000 men (*The Lancet,* February 20, 1993).

Researchers found that the likelihood of prostate cancer increased with the length of time since the operation. They speculate that the cancer may be triggered by the reduction in the secretion of prostatic fluid that follows vasectomy, or that the immune system may be compromised by the operation and, therefore, less able to ward off cancer.

Transplants

Bone marrow transplants—often used to treat leukemia and other malignant diseases—dramatically increase the risk of cancer. The risk can increase by as much as 8.3 times for people who have survived the transplant for 10 years or longer, while children who had transplants before they were 10 face the greatest risk of all.

Overall, the risk is greater, the younger the patient when he had the transplant. Researchers feel the risk may be linked to the amount of radiation therapy the patients received before having the transplant.

The research team, from the National Cancer Institute at Bethesda, Maryland, which produced these results, studied the records of 19,229 patients given bone marrow transplants between 1964 and 1992. They found that 80 had developed a new cancer, compared with an expected 29.8 cases from the general population (*New Eng. J. Med.*, 1997; 336: 897-904).

STRESS

Breast cancer link

Major stress—possibly sparked by a bereavement, a job loss or divorce—can cause breast cancer. Risks of developing breast cancer increase by almost 12 times if a woman has suffered stress in the previous five years.

Surprisingly, women who confront problems and try to work them out are three times as likely to suffer breast cancer as those who have an emotional response to their troubles.

Other risk factors, but ones considered of lesser importance by the researchers, included smoking and being postmenopausal. They found no evidence to suggest that environmental factors had any significant part to play.

This is a landmark piece of research because it is the first time researchers have been able to scientifically prove what many have suspected for a long time.

A team of English and Chinese psychiatrists, radiologists, surgeons and cancer specialists, led by Dr. C. Chen from the National Cheng Kung University Medical School in Taiwan, interviewed 119 women, aged between 20 and 70, who had been referred to King's College Hospital in London with a suspicious breast lump.

By questioning them, and assessing stress levels and other factors, they were able to show that women were more than three times as likely to develop breast cancer five years or less since suffering stress. This figure leaped to 11.6 times when adjustments were made for other factors such as age and the menopause (*BMJ*, December 9, 1995).

NUTRITION

There is no doubt that diet has one of the greatest roles in causing—or preventing—cancer (see p 149). Numerous studies have shown that too little or too much of certain nutrients can play a role in causing disease.

Cervical cancer

For instance, certain nutritional deficiencies can boost the chances of developing cervical cancer in a woman already at risk of the disease.

According to a multi-departmental study at the University of Alabama at Birmingham, US women deficient in folic acid were more likely to develop cervical abnormalities if other risk factors—number of sexual partners, use of the Pill, smoking or infection with human papillomavirus infection—were present. In particular, a low level of folic acid increased a woman's chances of developing cervical abnormalities by five times (*Journal of American Medical Association*, January 22/29, 1992).

Vitamin K

Vitamin K—often routinely given to newborn babies—has been linked with some childhood cancers. Newborns have extremely low levels of vitamin K—which helps with blood clotting—in their blood or stored in their liver. Doctors believe that unless vitamin K levels are artificially raised, babies could be at risk of developing potentially fatal vitamin K deficiency bleeding, also known as hemorrhagic disease of the newborn (HDN).

Those considered most at risk include premature babies, those having forceps delivery, "difficult" cesarean sections, those with liver disease or those born to mothers taking anticonvulsant or other medication which inhibits blood from clotting.

Conventional wisdom has it that exclusively breastfed babies risk vitamin K deficiency because breastmilk is low in in this nutrient. According to active birth pioneer and primal health researcher Michel Odent, this is only half right. True breast milk is low in vitamin K, but colostrum, which is secreted for a few days after birth, is very rich in vitamin K. One reason that babies suffer from HDN, he suggests, is that they are not put to the breast immediately after birth. In many parts of the world, hospitals still advise mothers to dispose of colostrum until the "real" milk comes in.

The widely reported study by Dr. Jean Golding, conducted at the Institute of Child Health in Bristol, England (the results of which were reproduced by Golding in a later study), show that babies receiving intramuscular (injected) vitamin K were twice as likely to suffer cancer as those receiving none (BMJ, 1992; 305: 341-46). This increased risk translates into 1.4 extra cases of cancer per 1,000 children by age 10.

All babies have a risk of HDN of 0.0086 percent. However, according to Golding's research, giving your child a vitamin K shot increases his cancer risk to 0.14. In other words, by injecting vitamin K, your baby may be 16 times more likely to get cancer than he was to get HDN.

Although the Golding results have not yet been reproduced anywhere else, and population studies in the US and Denmark have failed to find an increase in childhood leukemia after widespread use of injected vitamin K, there are several plausible theories as to why it may pose a cancer risk.

Golding and her colleagues pointed to experiments showing changes in chromosomes with high concentrations of vitamin K. Animal studies have also shown chromosome damage after vitamin K injections. Or, the cause may not be the vitamin per se, but another of the components that make up the injectable preparation, which could react with the vitamin to cause cancer.

Another experiment they cited suggested that a slight deficiency of vitamin K could actually protect against tumor growth. Or it could be that an injection itself is the problem, because it exposes newborns to foreign substances like viruses, which may trigger cancer (*BMJ*, May 16, 1992).

High-fat diets

Besides inappropriate doses of nutrients, the wrong ratio of fats, carbohydrates and proteins can predispose you to cancer. Scientists have proved a link between high-fat diets and colon cancer, for instance, an association long-suspected by researchers. Molecular scientists are discovering a complicated interaction between genetic and environmental factors which causes colon cancer, and which may point the way to other malignancies as well. It would also explain why some members of the same family, presumably eating the same diet, are more susceptible to cancer than others.

Scientists from the Jefferson Cancer Institute in Philadelphia have discovered that the difference may lie in "modifier" genes, whose interaction with mutant genes can determine whether someone will develop cancer or not. The modifier genes were found to be identical to a gene that instructs intestinal cells to produce an enzyme involved in fat digestion. The scientists suggested that high levels of this enzyme in the intestine in some way counter potentially harmful effects of dietary fatty acids.

Scientists have also discovered that other cancers—such as lung and bladder—have patterns of repetitive so-called "junk" DNA, which may serve as a marker for malignancies (*JAMA*, August 2, 1995).

CLOTHES

Even the clothes on your back—or front—may be linked with cancer. Tentative links have been made between cancer and some of the newer man-made fabrics or those treated with chemicals.

Bras

Wearing bras has been linked with breast cancer. Two medical anthropologists have concluded that women who wear a bra for 12 hours or longer every day are 19 times more likely to develop breast cancer than those who wear one for less than 12 hours. And women who wear a bra virtually all the time, even to sleep in, are 113 times more likely to develop cancer as women who wear theirs for less than 12 hours a day.

Sydney Ross Singer and Soma Grismaijer base their controversial findings on interviews with 4700 women from five US cities. The reason, they believe, is due to the way a bra artificially restricts the lymphatic system from flushing accumulated wastes from the body, which causes toxins to gather in the breast tissue. This, in turn, forms a breeding ground for a host of health problems, including cancer (*Townsend Letter for Doctors*, February/March, 1996).

Dr. Robert Blomfield of Hebden Bridge, West Yorkshire—a *What Doctors Don't Tell You* reader—has been suspicious of this connection for many years. He advises women to wear cotton bras, as he thinks it may be synthetic material that compounds the problem: "I have written to the Imperial Cancer Research Fund about this. Unfortunately, I was informed that the ICRF has no intentions of carrying out any research," he says.

Pyjamas

The American Government has banned the sale of pyjamas that contain Tris, a fire-retardant chemical, after it was found to cause kidney cancer in animals.

Although we don't know if the chemical can cause cancer in children, we do know that children are absorbing it through their skins. One doctor found high levels of Tris in children's urine and fat cells, even when the pyjamas had been washed several times.

Up to 51,000 American children could be carrying Tris in their systems and while none has yet gone on to develop cancer, the chemical tends to be very slow-acting (*Townsend Letter for Doctors*, June 1996).

2

Detection

Hiding Behind Screens

Medicine would have us believe that universal screening programs—by catching the disease "in time"—will prevent cancer. This notion is all the more seductive because various cancers among women are reaching epidemic proportions.

At the moment, women are the primary targets of these regular tests, mainly for cervical and breast cancer, although there has been talk of prostate and bowel cancer screening programs for men. Although cervical screening and mammography have been in place for years in America, Britain has only recently begun wholesale breast and cervical cancer screening; from 1991, three-quarters of eligible groups had been screened. However, behind publicly-voiced confidence in screening lies privately-admitted doubt.

Despite all the money being poured into massive

45

screening campaigns, no screening program anywhere is having the slightest impact on cancer mortality. In fact, because of the high potential for false positive readings—where people are told they have cancer when they don't—screening may only be increasing the number of patients mutilated through unnecessary drug treatment or surgery.

The medical literature has been awash with studies on both sides of the Atlantic demonstrating that some screening campaigns have no value. A study, from the University of British Columbia in Vancouver, even recommends junking mammograms altogether. They came to their conclusion after studying all the earlier trials claiming a 30 percent reduction in deaths from breast cancer for women over 50 who've been screened. This 30 percent risk reduction has been adopted as a mantra by the medical profession. It has been used to justify screening of other groups, such as women under 50, where no benefit has ever been shown.

Medicine's blind faith in screening was neatly illustrated by "Minerva", a columnist in the British Medical Journal, who cheerily admitted that there is "little hard evidence" but plenty of "sound reasons" for believing that screening for those over 65 is useful.

As age is the most important risk factor for the disease, and 65-year-olds may go on to live another 12 years, she figured, it's *got* to be good for them (*BMJ*, May 8, 1993).

There has been far less publicity, the Canadian researchers remind us, of all the studies that have been done since those early days, showing that mammography does no good for anyone in any age group, but does great harm through false positives and get-in-there-early intervention.

"Since the benefit achieved is marginal, the harm caused is substantial and the costs incurred are enormous, we suggest that public funding for breast cancer screening in any age group is not justifiable," the epidemiologists concluded.

It's hard to get any more damning than that. Or than the Bristol study of a quarter of a million women, showing that cervical screening is a dangerous waste of time.

CERVICAL SCREENING

The most widespread screening test is the Pap smear, so called after Dr. George Papanicolaou, who first developed it. In 1941, Papanicolaou and a colleague published a study demonstrating that malignant changes in the cervix could be diagnosed by examining cells taken from the vagina.

This simple, relatively painless test involves scraping a small sample of tissue from the neck of the womb and analyzing it for unusual cells. It was first adopted in various Western countries after publication of results from the pilot screening program in British Columbia showed that it was having an impact on lowering mortality.

Under Britain's current screening program, some three million smears are performed every year at an estimated cost (if doctors, nurses and lab time is included in the total) of £10 to £30 per woman screened.

Although there wasn't an overall national Government policy until recently, most doctors in the UK regard cervical cancer screening as part of standard good practice, recommending that all women between the ages of 20 and 65 repeat the test every three to five years. An article in *The Lancet* (January 13, 1990) recommended that screening be extended to women over 65, now considered a high risk group.

There is now a financial incentive for doctors to persuade women to have regular smears. If more than 50 percent of the women on their lists receive the tests, they are paid a bonus; the bonus is tripled if 80 percent take it.

Of course, no one would quarrel with the benefits of a simple, painless, risk-free test that promises to eradicate a common killer of women, *if it actually worked*. The problem is there is no convincing evidence anywhere to suggest that it does.

Professor James McCormick of the Department of Public Health at Dublin's Trinity College, an expert on mass screening tests, studied much of the available medical literature on the subject. He concluded: "There is no clear evidence that this screening is beneficial, and it may well be doing more harm than good" (*Lancet*, July 22, 1989).

By harm he means that many thousands of women are being subjected to risky treatments that could affect fertility or worse for a condition they do not have or which might right itself if left alone. The smear test has also never been proven to save lives in any country where it has been introduced. In fact, every study shows that it is making virtually no impact. The only area in Canada where screening has been universally adopted is British Columbia; nevertheless, the death rate of cervical cancer there matches the death rate of the rest of the country (*Mod. Med., Can.* 1973; 28: 6067-9).

In the UK, the annual death rate from cervical cancer fell before the test was introduced and has stubbornly remained at 2000 (although lately, the Government has said that the annual figure has dropped by 300).

In the UK and the US, mass screening programs,

like the National Cervical Screening program, have been mounted without a consistent nationwide policy about when or whom to screen, or how to follow-up abnormalities. Every large study of the program has revealed a decided lack of consistent standards.

Mounting evidence suggests that the smear campaign may be based on a faulty assumption: that abnormal, or "precancerous", cells on the cervix lead to cancer. The assumption has been inferred from two facts: cervical cancer progresses slowly and, if caught early enough, can be cured.

There are four categories of abnormal lesions, or "cervical interstitial neoplasia": CIN I, II, III and cancer. What we don't know is whether the early lesions —those in the CIN I and II categories—will go on to develop cancer. Professor McCormick cites a study published in the British Medical Journal examining the accuracy of cytology (cell) screening. The study demonstrates that some 10 percent of women screened have cervical abnormalities, "most of which," he notes, "would not progress to cancer" (*Follies and Fallacies in Medicine*, Tarragon Press, 1989).

Medicine doesn't really understand the usual progression of this kind of cancer—something it has tacitly begun to admit. Some cervical cancers appear to regress if left alone, while others progress so rapidly that the three-to-five year gap recommended by most screening programs would fail to pick them up in time. On this fragile foundation, women with an abnormal smear are frightened and stigmatized by the term "precancerous" when no one knows whether it is appropriate or not.

A 1988 study showed that nearly half of smears with mild abnormalities reverted to normal within two years. None of the patients developed invasive cancer during long-term follow-up (*BMJ*, 1988; 297: 18-21). A recent Canadian study showed that simple inflammation of the cervix may throw up an abnormal smear.

Besides the problem of not understanding the significance of results, the test is also so inaccurate as to be virtually pointless. There is no guarantee that a Pap smear will pick up the fact that you have cancer and there is a fair likelihood that you will be given a false positive—that is, told you have an abnormality that doesn't actually exist. In one study (published in *The Lancet*, January 13, 1990), the authors admit to false negative rates of between seven and 60 percent.

The conventional treatment for early "precancerous" lesions employs a colposcopy (a magnifying glass with light) and biopsy, diathermy (burning the abnormal cells) or cyotherapy (which employs a freezing probe to freeze the outlaw cells). These procedures can all cause hemorrhage or permanently damage the cervix resulting in an "incompetent" or narrowed cervix, and thus affect a woman's chances of carrying a baby to term.

Cervicography

Some quarters are quick to promote cervicography as an alternative to the Pap smear. The technique involves having your cervix painted with a weak solution of vinegar, which will stain any abnormalities white, after which a photograph—a cervigram—is taken.

Although initial reports show the technique is more accurate than the Pap smear, other reports says that this is only because the test produces even more false positives than the pap smear. Cervicography was shown to have a failure rate of 10 percent in a study performed at London's Marie Stopes clinic (*British Journal of Obstetrics and Gynecology*, March 1991). It also came up with abnormalities in 19 percent of the 1162 women tested, compared with 1 percent of those receiving routine smear tests. Dr. Elizabeth Hudson, President of the British Society for Clinical Cytology, said the method had been ruled out for mass screening because of a high rate of false positives.

MAMMOGRAMS

The other area of screening being stepped up sharply is mammograms, an x-ray of the breast designed to pick up early malignancies.

Breast cancer, the number two cancer killer after lung cancer, claimed the lives of an estimated 46,000 American women in 1993, the latest year that figures are available. England and Wales, though, have the worst breast cancer death rates of 50 Western nations, with 29 per 100,000 of the population dying from the disease.

In America, Congress responded to pressure by breast cancer activists by ordering the National Institutes of Health to increase spending on breast cancer by nearly 50 percent—to some $132.7 million. In the UK, the Government launched its National Breast Screening Program in 1990, offering mammography to women aged 50-64, and in its first year exceeded its target of screening 70 percent of the million women invited to participate every three years.

The American College of Obstetricians and Gynecologists also has called for more mammograms among women over 50. However, constant screening still can miss breast cancer. Mammograms are at their poorest in detecting breast cancer when the woman is under 50 and when the time between screenings is about two years.

Equally worrying, the test is also poor at detecting cancers in women who have a family history of breast cancer, possibly because of rapid tumor growth.

Researchers from the University of California confirmed the doubts that several international health boards have about the benefits of screening among the under-50s. The research team believe that mammograms are better at detecting cancerous growths in the over-50s because their breasts are more fatty. But their other findings, made after studying the records of 28,271 women aged over 30, give greater cause for concern. Paradoxically, those at highest risk because of their family history seem to be helped least by mammography (*JAMA*, 1996; 276: 33-8).

Following the results of a Swedish overview, which pooled results from five studies covering some 300,000 women, the medical establishment has adopted as gospel its results that for women 50 and over, regular screening can reduce breast cancer mortality by 30 percent. However, it is also generally agreed that no studies have shown a benefit for women younger than 50 (*Lancet*, 1993; 341: 1509-11).

Top breast cancer specialists Ismail Jatoi and Michael Baum from London's Royal Marsden Hospital, wrote a special feature labeling American doctors giving mammograms to the under 50s "negligent" because it can often do more harm than good (*BMJ*, 993; 336: 1481-3). But even among the over 50s, there is no conclusive evidence that mammographic screening is doing any good.

In the much quoted Swedish overview, the researchers came up with their figure by pooling all the results of three bands of age groups—the 40-49 year olds, 50-69 year olds and 70-74 year olds—into an overview. Although the study showed a positive benefit (29 percent reduction in mortality) among the 50s, there was no significant benefit among the 40 year olds or the 70s.

But findings from another Swedish study provide a potent argument against the recommendation of the Swedish health authorities that all women aged between 40 and 74 years should be screened between every 18 months and two years (*BMJ*, 1996; 312: 273-6). The cost of treating women who have had a false positive result (detecting cancer where there is none) is a third of the cost of providing screening for all women, they discovered.

Research has never before looked into the anguish, and the cost, involved for the women wrongly told they have breast cancer. Researchers from South Hospital in Stockholm monitored 352 women who had false positive readings. They made 1112 visits to doctors, had 397 biopsies, 187 follow-up mammograms and 90 surgical biopsies before being pronounced clear of cancer. Even after six months, only 64 percent had been given a clean bill of health.

The process cost £250,000, and women under the "danger age" of 50 accounted for 41 percent of these costs.

Researchers point out that these costs, extrapolated out, account for a third of the total cost of providing screening in the first place.

When you actually examine the statistics and science behind them, the original Swedish overview is the only study to show clear benefit, even among the 50s. The 30 percent improved survival figure being bandied about by medicine may also derive from several articles which have looked at all the studies of screening; although most studies did not show a clear benefit, the articles concluded that those that were most scientific, or "randomized" (that is, women assigned randomly to either screening groups or controls), all proved benefit (*BMJ*, 1991; 302: 1084).

However, James McCormick and the late Petr Skrabenek, scourges of unproven medical practice, point out that three of the four randomized, controlled trials "failed to reach statistically significant benefit for women aged 50 and over" (*BMJ*, 1991; 302: 1084).

Because we know that survival from breast cancer correlates with the size of the tumor, the rationale for screening is that the earlier you catch it, the smaller the tumor will be, and hence the greater your chances of beating the disease. However, Johannes Schmidt, an epidemiologist in Switzerland and long-standing critic of mammography, says that this rationale doesn't take into account that cancer doesn't always grow at the same rate (*Lancet*, 1992; 339: 810).

The Lancet admitted in a no-holds barred editorial that, despite all the treatments and screening, the number of women dying from the disease refuses to go down: "Let us stop complaining that screening ought to work if only we tried harder and ask why this approach is so disappointing," it said (*The Lancet*, February 6, 1993).

One reason may be that mammograms actually increase mortality. In fact numerous studies to date have shown that among the under-50s, more women die from breast cancer among screened groups than among those not given mammograms. The results of the Canadian National Breast Cancer Screening Trial published in 1993, after a screen of 50,000 women between 40-49, showed that more tumors were detected in the screened group, but not only were no lives saved but 36 percent more women died from

57

breast cancer in the group first offered screening (*Can. Journal of Public Health,* 1993; 84: 14-6). Similar results occurred in three Swedish studies and also in those conducted in New York.

This higher mortality figure may reflect the fact that mammography is indiscriminate, picking up many cancers which would do no harm if left alone. Schmidt suggests as much when he points out that mammography increases the incidence of breast cancer by one-quarter to one-half. This has two implications: the first is that these excess cancers, which are found to be benign, actually improve the survival statistics among the screened population of a test. Schmidt also estimates that mammography is 10 times as likely to pick up a benign cancer (and probably overtreat it) as prevent a single breast cancer death.

In one study at the Departments of Radiology and Surgery at the Brighton and Women's Hospital at Harvard Medical School, of 1261 cases only 26.1 percent of the mammograms recording some abnormality were found to be malignant tumors; at other radiology departments referring patients to the Harvard centre this figure was even worse—an average of 16.7 percent.

Dr. Michael Swift, chief of medical genetics at North Carolina University, demonstrated in a study of 1600 that moderately strong x-rays raised the risk of breast cancer five or six times in women who carry a certain gene, occurring in about 1 percent of the population, or about one million or more American women. Women (with the ataxia-telangiectasia gene) says Dr. Swift, have an unusual sensitivity to radiation and could develop cancer after exposure to "appallingly low" doses. He estimates that in the US, 5000 to 10,000 of the 180,000 breast cancer cases diagnosed each year could be prevented if women with the gene were protected from exposure.

Besides a genetic susceptibility, the physical trauma caused by mammograms could help to spread cancer. Mammograms use 200 newtons of compression, the equivalent of 20 one-kilogram bags of sugar per breast. Some of the modern foot pedal-operated machines are designed to exert a third again as much force—30 bags of sugar's worth of force, necessary in order to get the best quality image while keeping the radiation dose to a minimum.

A number of researchers, lately those from the Royal Jubilee Hospital in Victoria, British Columbia, speculate that compression during mammography can rupture cysts and disseminate cancer cells. This phenomenon has been observed in animal studies; if a tumor is manipulated, the spread of the tumor to other parts of the body can increase by up to 80 percent (*Ultrasound Med. Bio.*, 1979; 5: 45-9).

Nevertheless, there is huge resistance to change. A Swedish district that ended breast screening was forced to reintroduce the procedure, following immense pressure from the medical establishment.

Alvsborg County Council felt the costs of a mass screening program far outweighed any benefits, and that the money saved could be better spent helping those diagnosed with cancer. The council voted for the ban, following advice from the county's chief physician, Dr. Christer Enkvist, who felt that the advantages of screening are "extremely marginal" and can lead to unnecessary surgery.

Enkvist was pilloried in the Swedish press, and doctors and opposition political parties launched a campaign to have the decision reversed.

The Alvsborg councillors commented about their decision: "We realized it was a mistake." But was the mistake more political than medical? (*The Lancet*, March 23, 1996 and *BMJ*, March 9, 1996).

BIOPSIES

Biopsies—a procedure for investigating a suspect lump found on mammography—have their own set of problems. A thick needle is inserted into the breast under local anesthetic to remove a small piece of tissue. This is then examined for cancerous cells. In one study of 104 women undergoing biopsy, a quarter had problems afterward with the wound left by the needle such as infection or hematomas (*Lancet*, 1992; 339: 128).

Fine-needle aspiration, which can be done on an outpatient basis, has been served up as a less invasive alternative, when a lump has been found; in this instance, a fine needle with a syringe is inserted in the breast to draw out a specimen of the lump's contents. However, doctors have been known to puncture the lung causing pneumothorax (in which air enters the chest causing the lung to collapse). In 74,000 fine needle aspirations of the breast, this occurred in about 133 patients, or 0.18 percent (*BMJ*, 1991; 303: 924).

BREAST ULTRASOUND

With doubts growing about mammograms and other forms of x-rays, researchers are turning to mammary ultrasound. Ultrasound employs sound waves to produce an image on a screen.

As the instruments, including the transducer (the gadget producing the sound and "listening" for returning echoes), have grown far more sophisticated, ultrasound use has dramatically increased. These days, it is used to diagnose heart problems, a variety of tumors, circulatory problems, and to examine organs and body parts, including liver, spleen, uterus, placenta, brain and now breasts.

However, the success of ultrasound largely depends on the skill of the operator, as images can be hard to read and are open to misinterpretation. In particular, operators worry about visualizing "artifacts"—that is, a ghosted image of something that isn't there or mistaking something quite normal for something sinister. For instance, fetal hair has been mistaken for serious neural tube defects; bladders have been mixed up with pelvic tumors. This often happens when operators make errors in setting up scanning technique instruments or positioning the transducer (*JAMA,* March 6, 1991).

There's also the problem of false echoes creating images on the screen suggesting things that aren't there. This is a particular problem with curved, highly reflective surfaces such as the diaphragm or near large masses, such as the gallbladder or bladder. And problems in the accurate reflection of the sound beam can distort the size, shape, position and brightness of structures, making it possible to miss real problems.

With breast examinations, the most commonly used equipment is "real-time" high-resolution ultrasonography—which means you are seeing on the screen exactly what the transducer is picking up at that moment. Typically, a test requires at most 10 minutes of exposure. According to one study of 100 women with at least one breast nodule, the overall rate of accuracy of ultrasound was 74.8 percent. This, of course means, that in one in four cases, the diagnosis was wrong. In 10 cases, benign breast cysts were diagnosed as cancerous, and one breast cyst and one abscess were missed altogether (*Radiation Med.*, 1994; 12 (5): 201-8).

The other type of ultrasound used is color Doppler ultrasound, which measures the flow of blood, which in malignant tumors tends to be abnormal. There is no consensus on the accuracy of this technique. In one study, overall accuracy for detecting breast tumors was 82 percent (*Anticancer Research*, 1994; 14 (5B): 2249-51).

But in another large-scale study, the ability of Doppler color ultrasound to specify which type of tumor was only 46.9 percent (*Radiologia Medica*, 1994; 87: 28-35), and in a third, 83-100 percent of malignant tumors were correctly identified, but only 51-61 percent of benign lesions correctly identified (*Zentralblatt fur Gynakologie*, 1993; 115: 483-7).

The authors of one of the studies suggested that the color Doppler ultrasound be used only to add further information to that obtained with conventional ultrasound (*Radiologia Medica*, 1994; 87: 28-35). However, the technology does appear to be improving; presently the color method is used by comparing a color-spectrum analysis with surrounding tissue; in cancerous tumors, the color is typically more intense with sharp margins. In one study among 70 patients, this method only missed a single tumor (*Geburt und Frau,* 1994; 54: 432-6).

To date, the most accurate diagnostic method is combining ultrasound with "high speed" punch biopsies, once lesions have been identified by ultrasound. In one facility in Germany, this technique reached an accuracy rate of close to 100 percent (*Geburt und Frau,* 1994; 54: 539-44).

According to Professor William Lees, Director of Radiology at UCL Hospitals Trust in London, the best ultrasound should have Doppler as part of the system and use the two types in tandem, which will boost an operator's confidence about the accuracy of his diagnosis. Prof. Lees also believes that a skilled operator will have a much higher accuracy rate than the studies demonstrate—closer to 85 percent.

It may be that ultrasound has a similar overall batting average as mammograms. In one review of 80 patients with both benign and malignant lesions, mammograms picked up five cancers missed by ultrasound, but ultrasound discovered nine cancers missed by mammograms. In yet another study, ultrasound picked up four cancers that weren't yet palpable (*Ultraschall in der Medizin*, 1994; 15: 20-3).

At the moment, ultrasound isn't considered appropriate for screening, not only because of the error rate but because accuracy depends so heavily on skilled operators, and there aren't enough of them about. Prof. Lees agrees that it should not be used as a general-population screening tool, but may be a better first-line investigation of lumps felt during breast examination. When combined with a needle biopsy done on the spot, it can be highly accurate.

Dr. Alan McKinna, a consultant breast cancer specialist, says that most doctors don't like to rely on either ultrasound or mammograms alone, since ultrasound will pick up lumps you can feel but miss those you can't; mammograms will pick up the invisible lumps but may miss the big ones you can feel. Many doctors are using both.

The bottom line appears to be that ultrasound may be a better option than mammography to diagnose women with symptoms because it is safer and possibly more accurate than mammography for the under 50's. Although the technology is vastly improving and will probably eventually develop into a good tool, there are still some problems with accuracy.

SCREENING FOR OVARIAN CANCER

These days, most US gynecologists routinely screen for ovarian cancer. This widespread screening was prompted by the highly publicized death in 1989 of the American actress and comedienne Gilda Radner at the age of 42 from ovarian cancer. Screening involves ultrasound, pelvic examinations, and analysis of the blood.

However, this flurry of activity among doctors is against the express recommendations of the American government. The National Institutes of Health (NIH) recently recommended *against* routine screening, declaring that it is inaccurate and even dangerous.

The NIH said that these tests are so unreliable that surgeons have unnecessarily operated on many women who don't have the disease. Even if doctors do get it right, by the time the cancer shows up it's too late. And in only a quarter of cases is ovarian cancer detected at a stage early enough for effective treatment.

PROSTATE CANCER

With prostate cancer, medicine has been pushing routine screening of the over-fifties for the second major killer of older men. The three screening techniques include prostate-specific antigen (PSA), transrectal ultrasound (TRUS), and digital rectal examination (DRE). However, an analysis by the Toronto

Hospital in Ontario, Canada, concludes that high inaccuracy associated with these methods can do more harm than good. The main risk is unnecessary surgery, which causes widespread incontinence and impotence in a third of cases (*Lancet*, 1994; 344: 700-1). Furthermore, no evidence exists to show that men given a prostatectomy will survive any longer than those left alone and undergoing "watchful waiting."

One study discovered that 366 men given the all clear with a PSA test went on to develop prostate cancer, while raised values—which indicate the presence of the cancer—were found in just 47 percent of men who in fact had prostate cancer (*Jour. Amer. Med. Assoc.*, 1995; 273: 289-94).

Recently it has been discovered that the PSA can give false readings if the man has ejaculated in the previous two days. Men over 40 have very high PSA levels immediately after ejaculating, and though these start to fall significantly only six hours later, it takes 48 hours or more for the levels to normalize (*Urology*, 1996; 47: 511-16).

PRE-SCAN

These days, any doctor who detects a breast lump is likely to recommend a scan of some sort. According to *What Doctors Don't Tell You* columnist, Harald

Gaier, in the early stages, it's highly difficult to tell with absolute certainty whether a lump is cancerous or benign, unless the lump is biopsied.

Nevertheless, he says, it's possible to get some idea of the sort of lump it is by feel. Pain, changes in size during your menstrual cycle, easy mobility, absence of hardness and the presence of multiple nodules probably means there is no cancer, while malignant lumps are usually hard, irregular, non-tender and fixed.

A lump that remains the same throughout your cycle or increases dimpling of the overlying skin or tethering to the skin above or muscle below the lump is slightly more likely to indicate cancer.

Discharges, says Gaier, may indicate a number of things. A blood-stained discharge from the nipple could indicate cancer—or equally benign cystic mastitis. A greenish or yellowish discharge is invariably caused by mastitis; a watery one, early pregnancy; and a milky discharge (that is, if you're not breast-feeding), an adverse drug reaction.

Pain in the breast per se isn't necessarily cause for alarm (although it may sometimes prefigure the future development of breast cancer). Pain is often one of the collection of symptoms of PMS, and can be present with breast abscesses or a candida albicans yeast overgrowth.

Self-examination

Given the well-known inaccuracy of cervical smears, a better option may be your own observation. Professor McCormick says the most important early warning (early enough in most cases for treatment) may be any sort of bleeding between periods, for instance, after sex, or a persistent vaginal discharge.

The likelihood of cervical cancer increases with the number of sexual partners, smoking, taking the Pill or other estrogens, whether you've had any sexually transmitted disease or begun your sexual life early.

If you don't fall into any of these categories, be wary of your doctor pressurizing you into taking the test, particularly as he now stands to benefit financially from it.

If you do have to have a cervical exam, you might wish to ask for on a visual examination of the cervix rather than a routine smear. In a study of 45,000 women in Delhi, India, visual exams picked up nearly three-quarters of the cancers found among the sample size, by means of cervical erosions which bled on touch, small growths or, in general, a suspicious looking cervix (Singh et al, *BMJ*, 1992; 304: 534).

As for mammograms, medicine in general has downplayed the importance of regular physical examination of breasts as a diagnostic tool, despite an advisor to Britain's Chief Medical Officer admitting that "more than 90 percent of breast tumors are found by the women themselves." A seven-year study of 33,000 women by the Pennine Breast Screening Assessment Clinic in Huddersfield showed that self-examination could reduce breast cancer deaths by up to one-fifth. Although some lumps detected by mammogram aren't palpable, the reverse is true as well. Indeed, one researcher believes that routine screening lulls you into a false sense of security.

If you don't want a mammogram, make sure to opt for a regular program of self-examination (your doctor should be able to show you how) and breast examination by your doctor. If he is unwilling or has limited experience of physical examinations, you might ask to be referred to a clinic where these are routinely carried out, or find another doctor.

If you do decide to have a mammogram, shop around. Find out if the equipment to be used is dedicated—that is, specially designed for mammography and, therefore, able to give the best image with the least radiation.

Ask how many mammograms the lab does. The American College of Radiology recommends using a facility where each radiologist reads at least 10 mammograms a week. Machines should be tested at least once a year.

If a lump is found, either through mammography

or self-examination, you need to establish whether or not it is malignant. Some harmless cysts can be identified as such through a physical examination. If your doctor tells you it's a cyst but still suggests sending you for a biopsy, find out if it's really necessary.

If a lump is benign, returning each year for mammograms "just in case", is likely to serve only to create a problem where none existed. Dr. Ellen Grant, author of "The Bitter Pill", warns that a benign lump indicates that your anti-oxidation systems aren't working properly, possibly as a result of nutritional deficiencies. Radiation from repeated x-rays will only deplete your body's supply of anti-oxidating nutrients further, making cancer more likely.

Don't have a scan without a good reason—such as an abnormal breast exam. Although ultrasound appears to be safe, no long-term studies have been done in this area.

Preparing for ultrasound

Check that the operator is highly trained and highly skilled. Don't be shy about asking his accuracy rate or if there have been any serious cases he's missed.

Ask about the state of the equipment—how new it is, and when last serviced. Always seek out the best available equipment, specifically run by a radiologist specializing in ultrasound.

3

Conventional treatment

Does it work?

American cancer specialist Bernie Siegel argues in both his books, *Love, Medicine & Miracles* and *Living, Loving and Healing* (Aquarian), that the essential ingredient for healing is belief that the treatment is going to work. If the absolute certainty of healing is there, the road taken is secondary.

Siegel has seen "miracle cures" among those on chemotherapy and other conventional treatments. Often, these patients have been part of his Exceptional Cancer Patients program, an individual and group therapy which encourages cancer patients to express themselves through drawings, dreams and images. Nonetheless, many conventional treatments can come with serious side effects and, in this section, we outline what they can be.

It's worth noting the conclusions of the late Dr. Hardin Jones, professor at the University of

California in Berkeley. After analyzing cancer survival statistics for several decades he concluded in 1975 that "patients are as well, or better off, untreated." An extraordinary conclusion that has not only never been refuted but been upheld in subsequent research.

CHEMOTHERAPY

Chemotherapy is a drug-based treatment, usually taken orally or by injection, which attempts to shrink a cancer so that the diseased organ can be saved.

It was first proposed as a treatment for cancer right after World War II, when research on so-called mustard gas—cyclophosphamide—demonstrated that it has the ability to kill living cells, particularly those which rapidly divide, such as those in the intestinal tract, bone marrow and lymph system. Doctors soon came up with the idea that they could use mustard gas to poison cancer, which constitutes the most rapidly dividing cells of all. In fact, many of the drugs we use today are close cousins of mustard gas—one reason we find them so toxic (*The Immortal Cell*, Dr. Gerald B. Dermer, Avery, 1994).

It's probably no accident that medicine uses the tools of war against what medicine views as the most outlaw of cells. Nausea, vomiting and hair loss are the side effects most commonly associated with chemotherapy. However, these are only the beginning. Specific types of chemotherapy drugs bring their own particular shopping list of side effects. Cisplastin (Platinol), made of the heavy metal platinum, can damage nerves, kidneys, and cause hearing loss, seizures, irreversible loss of motor function, bone marrow suppression, anemia and blindness.

Mechlorethamine, an analogue of mustard gas (the "M" of MOPP treatment, the standard procotol for Hodgkin's disease), is so toxic that those administering the drug are advised to wear rubber gloves and avoid inhaling it. This drug is known to cause thrombosis, jaundice, hair loss, nausea and vomiting. Merck, its manufacturer, warns that "the margin of safety in therapy with MUSTARGEN is narrow and considerable care must be exercised in the matter of dosage. Repeated examinations of blood are mandatory as a guide to subsequent therapy."

A most dreaded complication of chemotherapy treatment is mucositis (or inflammation of mucus membranes, particularly of the gut and mouth), possibly leading to life-threatening infection (Cur. Op. Onc., 1995; 7: 320-4). Various types of chemotherapy can cause heart problems, destroy bile ducts, cause bone tissue death, restrict growth, cause infertility, lower white and red cell counts and lead to intestinal and lactose malabsorption (The Lancet, 1994; 343: 495).

In the early 1970s, medicine discovered that certain rare cancers would respond to chemotherapy and result in a person living longer. These include combinations of drugs for Hodgkin's disease, certain non-Hodgkin's lymphomas, some germ cell tumors, testicular cancer and certain cancers in children, such as Wilm's tumor, acute lymphocytic leukemia and choriocarcinoma, in which fetal cells transform into cancer and threaten the mother's life.

However, 25 years and many billions of pounds later, chemotherapy's modest successes are almost identical to what they were in 1971, says chemotherapy critic Ralph Moss (*Questioning Chemotherapy*, Equinox Press, 1995). The fact is, for most of today's common cancers, the ones that kill 90 percent of cancer patients every year, chemotherapy has never been proved to do any good at all and in fact may do harm.

After surgery, giving chemotherapy as a just in case measure to kill any "secret" pockets of cells has appeared to improve the survival prospects of certain groups of patients with breast, colon or lung cancer.

Recurrence rates are supposed to be reduced by a third and survival improved (*New Eng. J. Med.*, 1992, 326; 8: 563).

However, this evidence is only empirical (that is, based on observation, not scientific studies). It is very likely that it was the surgery alone that helped the survival of these patients.

Another side effect of chemotherapy, which is not so well reported, is the increased risk of developing leukemia. This is particularly so among women who receive certain forms of chemotherapy or drugs combined with radiation for breast cancer. One of its main problems is that it not only kills cancerous cells, but normal ones too, including those of the bone marrow—the foundation of the immune system—the intestinal walls and hair follicles.

The US National Cancer Institute in Bethesda, Maryland, studying 82,700 women diagnosed with breast cancer around the United States, concluded that the risk of leukemia was increased two and a half times after localized radiotherapy. Using alkylating agents alone increased the risk ten-fold; with combined radiation and drug therapy the risk increased by 17 times, and by 31 times with the chemotherapy drug melphalan, which was 10 times that of cyclophosphamide, another drug used to treat cancer.

There was little increase in the risk associated with cyclophosphamide doses of less than 20,000 mg. "Systemic drug therapy combined with radiotherapy that delivers high doses to the marrow appears to enhance the risk of leukemia," concluded the study.

An editorial in the same issue of the *New England Journal of Medicine* which published the study concluded that doctors need to be more "selective" in applying just-in-case therapy to breast cancer patients who have been cured (*The New England Journal of Medicine,* June 25, 1992).

Chemotherapy for cancer in childhood can also affect the fertility of men and women or cause birth defects. For men, drugs like procarbazine, chlorambucil and cyclophosphamide have been shown to be toxic to the testes; most male patients will be left sterile after a cumulative dose of 18 grams of alkylating agents like cyclophosphamide (although some men begin producing sperm again after 18 months).

For women, chemotherapy can cause ovarian failure and premature menopause—in virtually any woman treated, according to some studies (*CA-A Cancer Journal for Clinicians,* July/August 1990). This could be cause for concern, as 5 percent of cancer patients are under 34.

As for those who do go on to conceive children, a study conducted in New York found that of 202 pregnancies among 306 patients, 8 percent of the children of women and 7.9 percent of the children of the men had birth defects. Although this was not considered statistically significant, the study did show that congenital heart defects were identified in 10 percent of the children of women who'd been treated with dactinomycin, compared to 0.6 among a control population (*The New England Journal of Medicine*, July 18, 1991).

The leukemia risk was further endorsed by a study from Copenhagen's Department of Oncology of the Rigshospitalet. It showed that of 212 patients being treated with etoposide, cisplatin and bleomycin, five developed leukemia, which translates into a cumulative risk of nearly 5 percent from five to seven years after the start of the treatment. In the study, the cause was thought to be due to the etoposide alone or in combination with the other two drugs. It was also thought to be dose related, since all five patients had received a cumulative dose of more than 2000 mg/m2 etoposide, whereas no drug-caused cancers were found in those who had received less than that.

But, for all the risks of chemotherapy, does it actually work? A report by Dr. Ulrich Abel, a German epidemiologist, who published a small book entitled *Cytostatic Therapy of Advanced Epithelial Tumors—A Critique* (Hippocrates Verlag, Stuttgart), thinks not. Abel, who has a PhD in epidemiology and works in the Heidelberg/Mannheim Tumor Centre, examined virtually all the published literature dealing with chemotherapy—several thousand articles. He also wrote to some 350 cancer centers and experts around the world to find any other research that hadn't been published.

Abel concluded that the success of most chemotherapies was "appalling", that is, there is no scientific evidence for its ability "to extend in any appreciable way the lives of patients suffering from the most common organic cancer." Nor does it improve the quality of most patients' lives.

Dr. John Cairns of Harvard University's School of Public Health, says chemotherapy helps no more than 5 percent of patients. He also termed the chemotherapy used to treat malignancies too advanced for surgery, which constitute about 80 percent of all cancers every year, a "scientific wasteland" (*Lancet*, August 10, 1991 and *Townsend Letter for Doctors*, August/Sept 1991).

In one of the few reviews of all studies comparing chemotherapy against another form of treatment, chemotherapy proved no better than tamoxifen alone in women over 50 with breast cancer (*The Lancet*, 1996; 347: 1066-71).

Those cancers for which there is little evidence to support the use of chemotherapy include: breast, non-small-cell lung, colon and rectal, skin, liver and pancreatic and bladder.

Chemotherapy *has* been shown to increase the survival of patients with ovarian and small-cell lung disease, intermediate- and high-grade non-Hodgkin's lymphoma, and localized cancer of the small intestines although, again, this is not conclusively proven (*Current Op. Onc.*, 1995; 7: 457-65). Sometimes, these advantages are major, as with ovarian cancer, where it's been shown that it may extend the lives of patients for years. More often the effect is modest, as with lung cancer patients, increasing survival by only a few months (*Questioning Chemotherapy*).

Most cancer chemotherapy has been inadequately tested. Dr. Gerald Dermer, a cancer research scientist, claims that the first models for testing the cancer drugs were transplanted lymphomas in mice (that is, a tumor which has grown on one animal which is transplanted to another). Scientists also use man-made laboratory cell lines when experimenting with drugs.

However, Dermer discovered that cancer cells in both mediums are profoundly different than those in live human beings. Drugs that may kill transplantable tumors or cell lines have rarely been effective in humans (*The Immortal Cell*). The other problem is that cancer doctors define "cure" and "response" in different terms than you or I might. In the main, oncologists look only at "response"—that is, shrinking the tumor—as a measure of success, without considering whether it increases survival or improves quality of life.

Dr. Abel has found that when a tumor mass partially or temporarily disappears, those tumor cells which remain can sometimes grow much faster afterward. Often, patients who do not respond to chemotherapy survive longer than those who do (*Der Spiegel:* 1990; 33: 174-6, *J. Otolaryn,* 1995; 24: 242-52).

Ralph Moss describes a textbook on medicine, in which a top NCI scientist said that for most forms of cancer, many patients may initially respond. But in only three forms of cancer—ovarian, small-cell lung cancer, acute nonlymphocytic leukemia—did any appreciable percentage survive without disease, and even then it was, at best, less than a sixth of the total group of patients. In all the other types of cancer, disease-free survival was rare.

Shrinkage of solid tumors should not be overinterpreted, as it often has little or no survival benefit, according to oncology consultant G. M. Mead of the Royal South Hants Hospital (*BMJ,* January 28, 1995). Major chemotherapy manufacturer Bristol Myers discloses that only 11 percent of patients taking the carboplatin and 15 percent of patients taking cisplatin had a complete response to the drugs; remission lasted on average, about a year, and all patients survived, on average, only two years. Hardly a huge success, given that these are two of the most commonly used drugs for ovarian cancer—(which is supposed to be one of the types of the disease which responds best to chemotherapy (*Physician's Desk Reference*, 1995).

In the majority of studies, the most important question of all—does chemotherapy help you to live any longer than you would if you didn't get the treatment—is never even asked (*Questioning Chemotherapy*).

In the rush to be seen to be doing something about cancer, the US Food and Drug Administration has now officially sanctioned that new drugs for cancer can be fast-tracked on the market so long as they show they shrink tumors. There is no need to show that they lengthen the survival of cancer patients (*BMJ*, 1996; 312: 886).

The latest treatments are termed "rescue", as in rescuing you from the brink of death. Doctors harvest bone marrow from the patient before administering high-dose chemotherapy. The bone marrow is then replanted in the hope that it will somehow rescue the patient from murderously low blood counts.

Says oncologist Dr. Albert Braverman (*The Lancet*, April 13, 1991): ." . . many medical oncologists recommend chemotherapy for virtually any tumor, with a hopefulness undiscouraged by almost invariable failure."

After the success treating Hodgkin's disease, with a cocktail of cancer-killing drugs and steroids, medicine has applied this protocol to all other types of cancer, even though there is no evidence that it does any good at all. In oncology, more is always considered better.

In non-Hodgkin's lymphoma, one such protocol, ProMACECYTA-BOM, uses 10 powerful chemotherapeutic agents, when there is no solid evidence that even a single agent significantly saves lives.

Now, we hear that children who are successfully treated for Hodgkin's disease are 18 times more likely later to develop secondary malignant tumors. Girls face a 35 percent chance of developing breast cancer by the time they are 40—which is 75 times greater than the average.

These findings are a crushing blow to a medical establishment that had been congratulating itself for Hodgkin's disease treatment, which it considered to be a model of successful therapy. Cure rates of over 90 percent have been achieved from chemotherapy and low-dose radiation.

The risk of leukemia increased markedly four years after the ending of successful treatment, and reached a plateau after 14 years, but the risk of developing solid tumors remained high and approached 30 percent at 30 years.

These findings, which mean all children successfully treated for Hodgkin's disease need to be carefully monitored for the best part of their lives, come from the Late Effects Study Group, based at the University of Minnesota. The group followed 1380 children treated for Hodgkin's between 1955 and 1986 to discover any major reactions after treatment had finished.

The risk of developing a secondary tumor increased in those who were older when they had the cancer treatment, with 74 percent of cancers occurring in those whose Hodgkin's disease was diagnosed between the ages of 10 and 16 years.

But the most worrying development was the vastly increased risk of breast cancer among the female patients. The level of radiation seems to be the deciding factor, although the age when Hodgkin's was diagnosed was also important. Sixteen of the 17 breast cancer cases occurred in patients who were aged between 10 and 16 when treatment first started (*New Eng. J. Med.*, March 21, 1996).

RADIOTHERAPY

Radiotherapy is sometimes used instead of surgery, where a tumor is inaccessible, but is more often another adjuvant therapy. It is far less common than chemotherapy, simply because there are so few centers that can administer radiotherapy.

Small doses of radiation are usually pinpointed to the diseased organ by using a radiation machine (although sometimes internal radiotherapy can be prescribed where a radioactive isotope will be placed inside the body, resulting in a hospital stay). Nearly half a million patients in the US were treated with radiation in 1990, making radiotherapy one of the most widely used treatments for cancer.

Radiation was first used in medicine by Marie and Pierre Curie, the well-known French pioneers, at the turn of the century. The radiation used to treat cancer is called "ionizing radiation" which affects rapidly dividing cells, like tumor cells.

A breakthrough in the 1920's meant that doctors didn't have to depend upon natural sources of radiation anymore. They could produce it themselves, artificially. X-ray doses could also be measured and, therefore, controlled.

High-energy radiation—Cobalt-60—appeared in the 1950s and was used to treat cancer deep inside the body without burning the skin. By the 1960's, a new invention called the linear accelerator appeared which produced even higher energy.

Radiation beams vary widely in the energy they produce, from about 100 kilo-electron volts (KeV) to 25 million electron volts (MeV). As a rule of thumb, the higher the energy, the greater is the depth of penetration. Low energy beams deliver their highest dose at the skin. Beams with 25 MeV achieve their highest dose at a depth of about two inches.The newest measurement is the Gray (Gy); one Gy equals 100 rads.

Radiotherapy, chemotherapy, or combinations of the two treatments, are used to fight tumors. Alternatively, surgery can be used as the first line of attack. However, there is no evidence anywhere that combining radiotherapy with chemotherapy and surgery produces substantial gain in overall cures (RCS Pointon, ed, *Radiotherapy in Malignant Disease*, Springer–Verlag, New York, 1991).

Evidence is now emerging which suggests that radiotherapy is not quite the wonder cancer treatment it was originally thought to be. Not only does it spread the cancer, rather than eradicating it, in some cases, it actually causes cancer in healthy cells.

Breast cancer patients may be at risk of developing lung cancer after radiation. In one study, of 31 patients who'd received radiotherapy for breast cancer, 19 went on to develop a lung cancer on average 17 years later—mostly in the lung on the same side as the breast that had been irradiated (*Med. Onc.*, 1994; 11: 121-5). Some oncologists believe that the lung is especially sensitive to radiation damage, either scar tissue or inflammation—which would tend to argue against high-dose radiotherapy for lung cancer (*Strahl und Onk,* 1995; 171: 490-8). Breast cancer patients also risk soft-tissue cancers of the breast (*Int. J. Rad. Onc., Biol., Phys.*, 1995; 31: 405-10).

For Hodgkin's disease, radiotherapy also poses a risk of breast cancer years later (*J. Gyne., Ob. et Biol . Repro.*, 1995; 24: 9-12). In rectal cancer, animal studies have demonstrated the descending colon may be especially susceptible to cancer caused by radiation, particularly after surgery where blood vessels are joined up (*Dis. Colon & Rec.*, 1995; 38: 152-8).

Side effects also multiply when chemotherapy and radiation are given together.

In cervical cancer, where radiation bullets are often inserted in the vagina, cervical smears performed later often show abnormalities, such as fibrosis, and damaged cells (*Diag. Cyto.*, 1995; 13: 107-19). What this means over the long term is anyone's guess.

Although doctors are experimenting with maximum doses on diseases proving intractable, in many cases, higher doses of radiation may only lower survival. In one study examining the longer-term effects of radiation for cervical cancer, survival and local absence of disease decreased with every additional day of treatment beyond 55 days, no matter how early or advanced the disease (*Int. J. Rad. Onc., Biol., Phys.*, 1995; 32: 1301-7).

Perhaps most worrying, radiation can be a slow-motion time bomb, where side effects only show up years later. For instance, major urinary tract complications on patients treated for cervical cancer are most prevalent in the first three years, but can show up any time for 25 years (*Int. J. Rad. Onc., Biol., Phys.,* 1995; 32: 1289-300). In children, growth and premature sexual development can occur with doses as low as 18 Gy (*Int. J. Rad. Onc., Biol., Phys.,* 1995; 31: 1113-21).

Delivered by machine or from radioactive implants, radiotherapy often carries with it a myriad of side effects, a large number of them serious. The most common is fatigue, which occurs in most patients who receive therapy to a large area of their body. The skin also reddens, rather like a sunburn. Hair loss in the treated area is common.

Radiation to the head and neck can damage the salivary or tear glands, and you're left with a permanently dry mouth or eyes. Radiation to the abdomen may cause nausea, vomiting and diarrhea (*Effects of Radiation on Normal Tissues,* Churchill Livingstone, New York, 1993). Injuries to bone marrow are common and this leads to a weakened immune system. The bones may be damaged and osteoporosis may occur.

Radiation also scars most of the tissues it hits. Each part of the body can only tolerate a fixed amount of radiation. Once a dose has been given, radiation shouldn't be given again.

In virtually every form of cancer, radiotherapy has caused other appalling damage, and a few studies give an indication of its high incidence. In one study, one-third of patients receiving chemotherapy and radiation after surgery for rectal cancer ended up with major complications (*Aus. & NZ. J. Surg.*, 1995; 65: 732-6). We've also discovered that administering radiotherapy after surgery appears to cause more side effects than giving it before an operation (*Eur. J. Cancer*, 1995; 31A(7-8): 1347-50).

With breast cancer, the most feared side effect is fibrosis, where the skin is scarred and damaged. Even when the scar tissue is cut out, the skin rarely heals properly (*Strahl und Onk*, 1996; 172: 34-8).

Radiotherapy can also cause problems with reconstructive surgery afterward. Some 42 percent of breast implants had problems with pain and poor fitting in women who'd been irradiated, compared with only 12.5 percent of those who hadn't received radiotherapy (*Plastic & Recon. Surg.*, 1995; 96: 1111-5).

With cervical cancer, patients can find they are incontinent after radiation therapy following hysterectomy (*J. Wound Ost. & Contin. Nurs.*, 1995; 22: 64-7). Urinary problems also afflict men given pelvic radiation (*Eur. J. Canc. Care*, 1995; 4: 158-65). In cervical and testicular cancer, treatment can cause a high percentage of infertility (*Blood Rev.*, 1995; 9: 93-116), although with men, fertility might be able to be preserved if the dose to the unaffected testis is reduced to less than 2 Gy (*Clin. Onc.*, 1994; 6: 377-80).

Furthermore, if similar doses are used on women when pelvises are irradiated, the percentage of women undergoing premature menopause or infertility is low (*Inter. J. Rad. Onc., Biol., Phys.*, 1995; 32: 1461-4). Nevertheless, half of women given radiotherapy for cervical cancer suffer sexual dysfunction (*Int. J. Rad. Onc., Biol., Phys.*, 1995; 31: 399-404).

Radiation can also weaken your heart and vessels around the heart, causing narrowing of the arteries (*Giorn Ital Di Cardiol*, 1995; 25: 877-84) and cause thyroid dysfunction in up to 45 percent of patients given it for throat cancer (*Clinic Otol*, 1995; 20: 254-7). In head and neck cancer, radiation also can injure the brain (*Am. J. Neuro;* 1991; 12: 45-62), possibly lowering the intelligence of children (*Childs. Nerv. Syst.*, 1995; 11: 340-5), and damage the hearing (*Am. J. Oto.*, 1994; 15: 772-80).

Another underappreciated problem is fractures in bones exposed to radiation. This occurred in 6 percent of patients with soft-tissue sarcoma (*Eur. J. Can.*, 1994; 30A: 1459-63). Patients whose pelvises are irradiated can suffer so much bone damage that they must undergo total hip replacement. But even this is not a satisfactory solution. In one study of 56 patients undergoing joint replacement after radiation damage, 52 percent had the hips loosen, probably due to the weakening of bones. Although surgeons can use reinforcement rings to hold the joints there, nearly a fifth still loosen. Patients are also at risk of infection (*J. Bone & Jt. Srg.* (Brit vers): 1995; 77: 847-52).

Bowel cancer patients given radiotherapy have a high risk of long-term incontinence and major disturbances in bowel function, particularly when treatment is combined with chemotherapy (*Ann. Surg.*, 1994; 220: 676-82).

Injuries caused by radiotherapy treatment invariably follow breast cancer surgery. And many of the women who have set up the British Radiotherapy Action Group Exposure (RAGE), after suffering catastrophic arm injuries caused by radiation therapy for breast or cervical cancer, probably didn't need the treatment anyway.

Radiotherapy damage has left some of RAGE's members with excruciating pain, dietary complaints and repeated corrective surgery. However, in spite of the horror stories and years of research, 50 percent of patients with cancer are treated with radiotherapy during the course of their disease.

As one article pointed out: "Technology has advanced with accelerated regime . . . and new radiotherapy treatments. Yet still we are no further forward in dealing with toxicity from treatment. The focus of research has been on developing new cures, and only now are questions being raised about the quality of life of patients having radiotherapy treatment" (*Eur. J. Canc. Care*, 1995; 4: 158-65).

LIGHT THERAPY

Photodynamic therapy is a technique that uses light to destroy tumors. The patient is injected with a marker substance which attaches itself to cancer cells and makes them sensitive to light. This makes it possible to detect the location of the tumor with great accuracy, and by applying high intensity light with a narrow band of wavelengths the cancer cells can be destroyed with no damage to healthy tissue. For internal cancers, surgery is needed to insert an optical probe which carries the light to where it is needed.

In the UK, the Cancer Research Campaign is supporting research into photodynamic therapy. A light source called the Paterson Lamp has been developed which reduces the cost of treatment by replacing the laser source used in US research. At present this lamp is being used to treat non-melanoma skin cancer.

IMMUNOTHERAPY

Immunotherapy, medicine's latest fad, holds that you can fight cancer by giving help to the immune system. Behind this theory is the belief that the immune system has a built-in mechanism for fighting cancer, just as it fights infections. However, no one has been able to find foreign antigens (foreign proteins) in tumor cells. Unlike viruses, tumor cells have the same antigens as normal cells, so the immune system cannot recognize tumors as different in order to destroy them.

Some of the treatments centre around interleukin 2, or IL-2, a growth factor which is cultured with a patient's lymphocytes, to transform them into killer cells. This is mainly being tried out on kidney and skin cancer patients, with little success *(The Immortal Cell)*.

One study of colorectal cancer patients given a "vaccine" against tumor cells appeared to prove beneficial, until the study was investigated by the Committee on Government Operations of the US House of Representatives and found to be unreliable *(The Immortal Cell)*.

Researchers are attempting to use heat shock proteins (HSPs) to develop vaccines that offer new opportunities for cancer immunotherapy. Pramod Srivastava, Professor of Immunology in the biological sciences department at Fordham University in New York's Bronx, has been studying the mechanism by which HSPs help bolster the immune system. Produced by almost every cell in the body under normal conditions, HSPs increase in number when cells encounter stress, such as a sudden increase in temperature (*JAMA*, 1995; 274: 4; 291).

However, a generation of research and development has yet to yield an effective immunotherapy for cancer. And, like chemotherapy, the latest immunotherapy regimens make patients extremely sick, so it's considered for only a selected handful of the healthiest patients.

SURGERY

Is it effective?

In the late 19th century, the response of surgeons to cancer was to cut away huge amounts of healthy tissue as an insurance policy that they had "got it all." In head or neck cancer, surgeons removed part of the jawbone; in breast cancer, they removed the breast, lymph nodes and most of the chest wall. If you had cancer of the pelvis or internal organs in the early part of this century, you might lose the entire lower third of your body.

Although these days the treatments are less mutilating, today's doctors have continued with the notion that every last cancer cell must be cut away.

This is why most cancer specialists fear, more than anything, a "local recurrence." This means the cancer has returned to the spot where it was first detected.

Although fewer doctors persist with mutilating surgery, and the efforts are afoot to adopt conservative surgery in many areas, doctors still employ complicated mixtures of chemo, radiation and surgery to ensure against the return of one single cell.

However, Dr. Richard Evans, an American surgeon, is one of the few with the courage to challenge this paradigm of all-out nuclear warfare. Dr. Evans, who scoured much of the medical literature about cancer, discovered that in many types of cancers, although conservative surgery without radiation or chemo does produce more local occurrences, patients don't die one day sooner than those who also get chemotherapy or radiation as well. In other words, he writes, "there is no survival disadvantage to leaving tumor cells alone and simply observing the patient."(*Making the Right Choice*, Avery Publishing, Garden City Park, NY, 1995). This is also the case with soft-tissue sarcomas—cancers of muscle or fat, and skin cancer. Dr. Evans cites studies demonstrating that when surgeons use slightly larger margins (1-2 cm) in excising certain types of tumors, patients live just as long as they might with chemo or radiation, but without the side effects or the dangers that the either treatment offers.

Surgery on its own can be the treatment of choice for certain early cancers: the stomach, colon, cervix, rectum, thyroid, skin, breast and testis. When conservative surgery is used, there is often no lessening in survival, so long as recurrences are promptly removed. For instance, in a randomized trial, when rectal-sparing conservative surgery was done, there was no difference in survival. Bowel function was preserved (*Ann. Surg.*, 1986; 204: 480-7).

Nevertheless, *"The Efficacy of Surgical Treatment of Cancer"* (*Medicinal Hypotheses*, 1993; 40: 129-38) and "The Efficacy of Surgical Treatment of Breast Cancer," (Ibid), show that there is no scientific evidence that surgery has any effect on survival or mortality for any form of cancer—which suggests that cancer must be a systemic disease.

The second paper analyzes the results of six randomized mammographic breast cancer screening trials which led to claims that mammograms save lives by providing earlier detection and, therefore, enabling earlier surgical intervention. This claim is rejected on the grounds that some of the trials were poorly conducted, which could have skewed the results. The papers' author—Don Benjamin of the Cancer Information and Support Society, Crowsnest, New South Wales—shows that the trials with the greatest number of easier tumors detected had the smallest reduction in mortality and those with the smallest number detected had the largest reduction in mortality—so surgery could not have produced the observed result.

Mastectomies

Most doctors still overtreat early breast cancer, cutting out more than they need to, or overload the patient with drugs or radiation. Despite a variety of surgical techniques, a host of back-up therapies and many confident headlines about breast cancer breakthroughs, the astonishing truth is that surgical treatment of breast cancer hasn't advanced one single step in the past century.

Dr. Edward F. Scanlon, of the Northwestern University Medical School, summarizes the prevailing view: " . . . over a period of 100 years, breast cancer treatment has evolved from no treatment to radical treatment and back again to more conservative management, without having affected mortality" (*JAMA*, September 4, 1991).

The standard procedure for breast cancer this century has been the radical mastectomy, a mutilating operation which involves removing the breast, much of the skin, the chest wall and the lymph nodes, developed by Dr. William Halsted a hundred years ago. Shortly after the Second World War, a study at three hospitals in Illinois showed little difference in five- and 10-year survival rates between radical mastectomies, simple mastectomies, or simple removal of tumor. In 1969, *The Lancet* (November 29) reviewed 8000 cases and again found no difference in survival between any of the procedures. Nevertheless, the Halsted procedure maintained its grip on the minds of most surgeons well into the 1970s and 1980s, when in some areas it was replaced by a modified radical mastectomy, which removed tissue and breast, but left the chest wall, or a simple mastectomy, which only removed the breast itself.

Like the earlier studies, numerous trials in the 1980s have shown that mastectomy provides no benefit in terms of cancer recurrence or survival over breast-conserving surgery (BCS), such as simple lumpectomy (removal of the tumor itself) or quadrantectomy (removal of a portion of the breast). In one, by the National Surgical Adjuvant Breast and Bowel Project in Pennsylvania, of nearly 2000 women over nine years, there was no significant difference in survival without the cancer spreading to other parts of the body between those who had undergone lumpectomy, lumpectomy plus irradiation, or total mastectomy.

New research from the National Cancer Institute in Bethesda, Maryland, and based on 247 patients, confirms that lumpectomy and radiation were just as effective after 10 years in controlling early stage (I and II) cancers (*NEJM,* April 6, 1995).

As a result of these comparative studies, the American National Institutes of Health (NIH) in 1990 recommended that surgeons opt for breast conservation surgery over mastectomy for the majority of women with stage I or stage II breast cancer. By this, they mean cancer less than 4 cm. in diameter limited to a single breast without involvement of the chest muscle or overlying skin. In the past, doctors felt that cancer found in the axillary lymph nodes was evidence that the cancer had spread, and grounds for radical mastectomy.

With the NIH's announcement, the involvement of the lymph nodes (so long as it is on the same side as the tumor) is now considered immaterial.

Regardless of the NIH's decision, most doctors don't offer BCS to the majority of women with early breast cancer. A Seattle study (*JAMA*, December 25, 1991) examined cancer registry information between 1983 and 1989. In total, less than a third of women with stage I or II disease were offered BCS. Furthermore, that proportion declined after 1985.

The Seattle study also found that doctors failed to offer radiation therapy to postmenopausal women and were more likely to recommend mastectomy to the older group than to younger women, even for the same stage of breast cancer. The more affluent and well educated the woman, the greater her chances of being offered BCS.

The lack of information or support by doctors for

BCS may account for the suspicion with which many women view breast-conserving measures. This point of view is epitomized in a letter written by Dr. Michael G. Sarr and others to the *JAMA* (August 19, 1992). "Many view mastectomy as dealing with the problem immediately and completely, without post-operative radiotherapy. The acceptance, indeed preference, of mastectomy over breast-preserving surgery by the majority of our patients . . . implies that these patients adjust readily to the loss of the breast."

Indeed, several noted cancer specialists have attempted to demonstrate that women given mastectomies suffer no more psychological trauma than those undergoing BCS. Noted breast cancer specialist Michael Baum and others from London and Manchester studied the psychological outcome of women given mastectomies versus those given BCS (*BMJ*, September 22, 1990). The study found that about a quarter of those given either operation were depressed or anxious, and so concluded that "there is still no evidence that women with early breast cancer who undergo breast conservation surgery have less psychiatric morbidity [illness] after treatment than those who undergo mastectomy." Significantly, the study found that patients treated by surgeons who allowed them to choose were less likely to be depressed than those whose decision was made for them.

Besides your education or ability to pay privately, where you live has a lot to do with whether you are offered BCS or mastectomy. Two articles in the *New England Journal of Medicine* (April 23 1992) showed a marked difference in the use of BCS in the US, depending on geographical area. Women were more likely to be offered BCS in the Northeast (17 percent) or Mid-Atlantic States (20 percent) than they were in the South (5.9-7.3 percent). BCS was more on offer in urban than rural areas, in teaching hospitals, large hospitals and those with onsite radiation therapy.

Interestingly, an editorial in the same issue pointed out that higher rates of conservation surgery were found in those 17 states with informed consent laws requiring doctors to offer patients with breast cancer information about their treatment options.

Besides the problem of overtreatment, too much surgery might delay your doctor's ability to discover whether the cancer has spread. Dr. Bernard Fisher and colleagues from the National Surgical Adjuvant Breast and Bowel Project in Pennsylvania, writing in *The Lancet* (August 10, 1991) about a nine-year study of 2000 women comparing mastectomy to lumpectomy, showed that mastectomy or radiation therapy actually prevented the diagnosis of distant disease since the recurrence of another tumor tended to be a "powerful" marker that the cancer could spread, thus aiding its early treatment: "These findings further justify the use of lumpectomy," concluded Dr. Fisher.

Although the results of this study were found to be falsified, independent teams and more recent evidence confirmed that lumpectomy is just as efficient as radical mastectomy in controlling cancer.

Cell spread

Certain forms of surgery have also been found to help spread the disease. Breast cancer tumors can spread during surgery. Surgeons who operated on 16 women found that six had more cancer cells circulating during the procedure. They also discovered a link between cell shedding and the density of the tumor.

The woman with the densest tumor had the greatest number of cells circulating during the operation (*The Lancet*, November 18, 1995).

Prostate surgery

Radical surgery to treat prostate cancer only succeeds in spreading the condition, new research has discovered.

Doctors had assumed that the poor survival rate after prostatectomy was because the disease was systemic like the other cancers. But researchers have discovered that the surgery itself can accidentally spread cancer cells to other parts of the body. They monitored 14 consecutive operations, and discovered prostate cells in the blood of 12 of the patients afterwards. Just three had tested positive before surgery.

Researchers have recommended that surgeons should use a surgical technique called "no-touch" when carrying out a prostatectomy (*The Lancet*, December 9, 1995).

Researchers have also concluded that prostatectomy patients tend to have a better survival rate if they have an open prostatectomy (OP) rather than a transurethral prostatectomy (TURP). After studying records of 13,815 men who underwent a prostatectomy between 1963 and 1985, they found there was a higher mortality rate among men one year after they had TURP, although there was an increased mortality rate with OP one month following surgery.

Researchers from the University of Oxford suggest that the mortality rate is not linked to either procedure per se, but probably to the general fitness of the patients (*The Lancet*, December 9, 1995).

Hysterectomies

In some 40 percent of hysterectomies one or both of the ovaries and fallopian tubes are removed as well. Conventional wisdom is that leaving a woman her ovaries after a hysterectomy is like leaving a cancerous time bomb inside her. This is not borne out by research. Among women who have ovarian cancer, only 5 percent will have had a prior hysterectomy. Looked at from another angle, only 0.2 percent of women who have a hysterectomy will go on to develop ovarian cancer (*Fertil Steril*, 1984; 42: 510-4).

Genetic susceptibility to ovarian cancer may be linked with susceptibility to other forms of intra-abdominal cancer. In one study where the ovaries of women genetically predisposed to ovarian cancer were removed as a just-in-case measure, more than 10 percent developed some other form of intra-abdominal cancer (*Lancet*, 1982; 2: 795).

Studies show that when a pre-menopausal woman's ovaries are removed, she will often experience severe menopausal symptoms (*Am. Jr. Ob. Gyn.*, 1993, 168: 765-71). Even if the ovaries are preserved after hysterectomy, they are prone to early failure, leaving a woman with menopausal hormone levels at a much earlier age (*Fertil Steril*, 1987, 47: 94-100).

Often there is no medical indication for removal of the ovary—some hospitals simply require it, as a matter of policy, when a hysterectomy is performed. Women are generally not told this, any women considering hysterectomy should be clear about what the policy at her local hospital is and go elsewhere if necessary.

It is wrongly believed that a woman's ovaries stop functioning in her mid 40s—often the rationale for oopherectomy in the older woman. Yet studies show that the older ovary continues to produce a hormone that, in menopausal women, is converted into estrogen in the fat deposits in the body, thus continuing to protect the heart and bones (*Fertil Steril,* 1984; 42: 510-4). Synthetic hormones do not do the job as well. The ovaries should be preserved at all costs.

OTHER DRUGS
Tamoxifen

Besides surgery, medicine has experimented with a number of anti-cancer drugs. Although there is no drug to kill off cancer completely, a number of hormone antagonists are supposed to stop hormone-dependent cancer from spreading.

The most popular of these is tamoxifen, for breast cancer. Hopes were pinned on this drug as a preventative in healthy women until the drug underwent a study in Scotland.

The Scottish researchers discovered that women who have taken the drug for up to 14 years face a greater risk of developing thromboembolism, when the blood vessel becomes blocked by a clot. Paradoxically, the drug also reduces the risk of heart attack, although researchers from the University of

Edinburgh warn that healthy women taking the drug should be carefully monitored.

Research in the US and the UK, also to test whether tamoxifen is an effective cancer preventative in healthy women, has been delayed following a rash of bad publicity surrounding the drug. As a result, few women were prepared to volunteer. A Swedish study, in 1994, revealed the drug could cause uterine cancer after long-term use, while later research also revealed a link with gastrointestinal cancer.

The American National Cancer Institute's (NCI) findings mirrored those from another Scottish study. NCI researchers found that women given daily doses of 20 mg of the drug for five years reported a 92 percent disease-free survival rate, as against 86 percent in patients scheduled to receive 10 years of tamoxifen therapy. Similarly, researchers from the Scottish trial reported a 70 percent success rate among women given the drug for five years, against 62 percent among those who took it longer.

NCI investigators were satisfied they had sufficient evidence: "The data, taken together with the results of the Scottish trial, provide no evidence of benefit for continuing tamoxifen beyond five years," they say (*The Lancet*, December 9, 1995).

Breast cancer death rates in England and Wales have fallen by 12 percent between 1987 and 1994.

However, health officials who have been congratulating their extensive mammogram screening programs as the reason for the sudden drop in breast cancer deaths need to think again. New research has discovered no evidence to link the two.

The National Cancer Registration Bureau believes the fall may be more likely associated with the increasing use of tamoxifen slowing cancer growth, than with any screening.

Aspirin

Doctors have also been experimenting with a number of other drugs to treat or prevent cancer. Aspirin, which is now being hauled out to treat everything from headache to stoke, is the latest cancer preventative.

The latest recommendation is that people at high risk from developing cancer of the rectum or colon should start taking between four and six aspirin a week. A low-dose aspirin regime—using 325 mg each time—could cut the risk of colorectal cancer by half in the long-term. Unfortunately, these benefits only start becoming apparent after 10 years of consistent use, and risks are halved only after taking aspirin for 20 years.

People who take aspirin run the risk of suffering stomach bleeding, but doctors say this is far outweighed by the benefits among high-risk groups, which include sufferers of inflammatory bowel disease, breast, ovarian or endometrial cancers, or a previous adenoma or large-bowel cancer. Others considered in a high-risk group are those whose family has a history of colorectal cancer.

These findings are based on the major Nurses' Health Study, which has tracked the health of 121,701 nurses in the US since 1976 who have a known or suspected risk of developing breast cancer or heart disease. Researchers discovered that the women who consistently took four to six aspirin a week from 1984 to 1992 halved the risk of developing the cancer, and the risk continued to fall as the dosage increased, although cases of bleeding were reported in women who took more than 14 aspirin a week. Women who took two aspirin a week only saw a noticeable reduction of risk after 20 years; after four years' usage at these levels, there was virtually no benefit at all.

Although the research involves only women, researchers say the same benefits should be experienced by men. Researchers believe that aspirin indirectly blocks tumor growth, although they also accept that other factors could have been at play and that more research is needed (*N. Eng. J. Med.*, September 7, 1995).

4

Alternative cancer treatments

What works?

Although many of the most promising alternative cancer therapies have been around for most of this century, there is a peculiar lack of scientific study assessing them.

This situation is more a comment on the orthodox camp's paranoia about employing any new treatment against cancer (and thus admitting defeat or letting go of a multi-billion dollar industry) than a statement about the efficacy of the treatment in question. Despite this climate of suppression, a number of alternative treatments have been the subject of some properly designed laboratory and clinical research. Although all would benefit from further study, they certainly appear more promising than most of the tools of orthodox medicine.

Cancer represents a healer's greatest challenge. It operates like an alien inside your body. Its biochemical laws are different from yours. It's able to completely disarm your immune system, in effect, creating an immunological shield to protect itself—all the while it fires out substances that weaken the integrity of your cells and reproduces out of all control.

Supposed cures have been almost as ingenious as the disease itself. For example, they range from the well-documented cases of Dr. Hugh Faulkner, who recovered from apparently terminal cancer by adopting a macrobiotic diet, to Norman Cousins who laughed his way to wellness by watching Laurel and Hardy movies at home.

In between are the thousands of cases who improved by taking vitamins, changing their diet, adopting meditational techniques or by finding some form of self-expression. The use of nutrition and vitamins have also successfully been used as treatments.

It bears repeating that the most important element to healing is a belief and certainty that your choice will work. Alternatives can be the preferred choice for those who want to play an active part in their own healing, rather than being a passive patient. *Special thanks are due to the American writer Richard Walters who helped compile some of this section from work originally done for The Townsend Letter for Doctors and Patients.*

Nearly 10 years ago, the American Government's Office of Technology Assessment published a report about the efficacy of alternative treatments. That report was widely denounced as biased and unscientific by many alternative patient groups and researchers alike in the field of cancer.

Alternative cancer therapies regard the tumor as a symptom. To the alternative practitioner, cancer is a systemic disease that affects the whole body. In holistic medicine, the body is a healthy, self-regulating organism which doesn't get sick unless something harmful is done to it. Instead of attacking the tumor, many alternative therapies aim to rebuild the body's natural immunity and strengthen its own ability to destroy cancer cells.

THE MOST PROMISING ALTERNATIVE TREATMENTS

Immuno-augmentative therapy

Dr. Lawrence Burton's Immuno-Augmentative Therapy (IAT) consists of injections of four blood proteins that augment immune system functioning and shrink tumors. Burton, former Senior Oncologist at St Vincent's Hospital in New York, astonished the medical world in 1966 when he and a colleague injected cancerous mice with a serum, causing the tumors to shrink by half in just 45 minutes. Ninety minutes later, the tumors had all but vanished. This unprecedented demonstration, made under ACS auspices in the presence of 70 scientists and 200 science writers, generated front-page headlines in major newspapers around the world. Burton repeated the demonstration months later before an audience of cancer specialists at the New York Academy of Medicine, this time in a controlled experiment, with comparable results.

Burton opened a cancer clinic in Great Neck, New York, in 1974, and treated many patients who reportedly experienced dramatic tumor shrinkage or remissions. Dr. John Beaty of Greenwich, Connecticut, who sent 20 advanced cancer patients to Burton, reported tumors regressing in 50 percent. Despite these results, Food and Drug Administration harassment forced Burton to close his clinic in 1977 and open one in the Bahamas.

In 1985, US health officials of the NCI and the Centers for Disease Control (CDC) falsley accused Burton's Bahamian clinic of using AIDS-contaminated serum on patients returning to the US. Under American pressure, the Bahamian Ministry shut down the clinic. It was only reopened when lawsuits were filed against NCI and CDC, and after Burton's patients appealed to members of the US Congress. These patients included the distinguished cancer surgeon Dr. Philip Kunderman (former Chief of Thoracic Surgery, Roosevelt Hospital, New York), who stated that his own cancer was successfully controlled on IAT.

One of the most promising cancer treatments today is tumor necrosis factor (TNF)—a blood derivative said to cause rapid tumor shrinkage. In the view of some observers, TNF came about as a direct result of Burton's original research.

Peptide therapy

Former Professor at Baylor College of Medicine, Texas, Dr. Stanislaw Burzynski, a Polish emigre physician (at 25, one of the youngest men in Europe ever to obtain an MD and PhD), developed a cancer treatment using peptides—building blocks of amino acids occurring naturally in human blood and urine.

His research points to a severe shortage of these substances, called antineoplastons, in cancer patients. In reintroducing the peptides into the patient's bloodstream—either intravenously, or orally with capsules—he found that they experienced tumor shrinkage or complete remission.

Harris Coulter described the role of peptides discovered by Burzynski as tantamount to discovering a "second immune system." Unlike our ordinary immune system, which protects us against foreign "invaders", this second internal system appears to guard against defective cells like cancer by "reprogramming" them to develop normally again. In Burzynski's view, this means that cancer is a disease of incorrect information processing, where the cell reproduction goes haywire. The antineoplastons (anti-cancer compounds) which correct this bad programming appear to be deficient in cancer patients. Burzynski began to extract these substances from blood, tissue and urine and developed a method of reintroducing them into the blood of people with cancer.

Unlike many cancer pioneers, Burzynski has published many of his findings, which have been confirmed by independent laboratories. He also has a five-foot stack of records and studies which he has submitted to the US Food and Drug Administration to attempt to get a "new drug" license, and he's passed the first phase of the FDA's clinical trials. In the supporting study, the antineoplastons showed good results in patients with prostate cancer, bladder cancer and brain tumors; many had complete or partial remissions and one-fifth survived at least five years. Many of his original patients, he claims, are healthy 13 years later (paper presented at the Fifteenth International Congress of Chemotherapy, Turkey, 1988). In another study for the FDA's second phase of trials Dr. Burzynski gave his antineoplastons to 20 patients with advanced astrocytoma (brain cancer). Four patients achieved a complete remission and two others, a partial remission. Since the study began in 1990, two more patients have achieved partial and complete remission respectively. (D. Adam, ed, *Recent Advances in Chemotherapy*, Futuramed Publishers, 1992).

In a paper delivered at the 1986 International Cancer Congress, the world's most prestigious forum on cancer research, Dr. Burzynski reported five-year follow-up results in a clinical trial of his methods with advanced cancer. Forty-seven percent of the patients experienced complete remissions, 60 percent had objective remissions and 20 percent survived over five years without cancer. Burzynski has published his results extensively in the peer-reviewed medical literature. Confirmatory studies at major US medical centers are part of a large and growing body of evidence that antineoplastons are effective in treating human cancer patients.

Although Burzynski applied for drug approval, FDA dragged its feet for six years, after which—on the same day Burton's clinic in the Bahamas was shut—agents raided his institute, looking for vague "violations" and seized all of his scientific, medical and personal records.

Although the FDA has now licensed Burzynski to administer his treatment at his own clinic in Texas, recently he was charged with violating laws of interstate commerce out-of-state (patients of his were simply ordering his medicine). He was later tried and acquitted of all charges.

Govallo immune therapy (VG1000)

For many years, Russian immunologist Dr. Valentin Govallo and his colleagues at the Immunology Laboratory in Moscow attempted to fight cancer by simply boosting the patient's immune system. However in the 1970s, Govallo discovered similarities between a fetus's "immunological shield"—which prevents it being attacked by its mother's immune system—and that of tumors, which similarly disable their host's defenses. Govallo described the ability as akin to a "burglar who first turns off the burglar alarm before he goes about stealing things." Govallo and his colleagues developed a means of suppressing the immune system of the tumor through a "vaccine"—called "VG-1000" using tissue from healthy human placentas harvested after live births. According to Govallo, if you can suppress the tumor's immunity, "even a dying patient can overcome the tumor." Dr. Govallo discovered that an extract of human chorionic villi, when added to a test tube of white blood cells, "effectively blocks all reactions of cell immunity" (*Cancer Chronicles*, 1994; 5: 3).

Since 1974, Govallo has treated approximately 100 patients. He has documented evidence showing that the 10-year survival rate for those with advanced cancer is about 60 percent (Govallo, *The Immunology of Pregnancy and Cancer*). Of 45 patients with advanced cancer treated in 1974, 29 are still alive—a survival rate of 64.4 percent. He says that VG-1000 is most effective against breast, lung, colon and, kidney cancer, malignant melanoma and brain tumors.

Currently, Dr. John Clement of the Immunology Researching Center in Freeport, Bahamas, and medical historian Harris Coulter, have developed a protocol for the scientific evaluation of VG-1000 with a clinical trial, which began in September 1996. Coulter emphasizes that VG-1000, like other immune therapies, works best in patients who have not been extensively treated with radiation or chemotherapy. Patients with metastastic liver cancer should not undergo this treatment; in one instance, a patient with this disease developed reactive hepatitis.

Gerson therapy
German-born Dr. Max Gerson's program is a low-fat, salt-free, meat-free diet including organically grown fresh fruits and vegetables and 13 glasses of freshly

squeezed juices daily, at hourly intervals.

Gerson famously realized more than 50 years ago that the high sodium-potassium ratio of the modern Western diet was riotously out of kilter. He also introduced detoxifying with coffee enemas, which stimulate the liver and large intestine into excreting toxic elements from the body.

A 1990 Lancet evaluation of seven Gerson patients with extensive metastasized cancer at Maudsley and Hammersmith Hospitals in England revealed that three patients were in complete remission. Patients also reported a high degree of control over the treatment, low pain scores and little requirement for drugs (*The Lancet*, 1990; 336: 667-8).

Other evidence about the success of Gerson therapy is decidedly mixed. In one 1995 study of patients with melanoma, every one of the stage I and II, and 82 percent of stage III patients survived for five years. Among those undergoing conventional treatment, only 39 percent with stage III disease survived for the same length of time (*Alt. Thera.*, 1995; 1: 29-37).

However, in a 1994 study of 22 patients, most with advanced disease who'd been unsuccessfully treated with chemotherapy, radiation and surgery, all died within an average of seven months. In another study of 18 patients, all but one died within nine months, even though less than half had had advanced cancer when they arrived at the clinic and six hadn't undergone any conventional treatment (*J. Nat. Med.*, 1994; 5: 745-6).

Coley's toxins

At the end of the last century, Dr. William Coley, a young New York surgeon, discovered that one patient with bone cancer had survived the cancer because he'd contracted an infection by *Streptococcus pyogenes*, a life-threatening skin disease. Coley spent the next 40 years refining what came to be known as Coley's toxins—using byproducts of *Streptococcus pyogenes* plus *Serratia marcescens*, which helps to intensify the activity of the first germ. What appeared to happen was that the patient's temperature and pulse rapidly rose—sometimes by six degrees. In the view of author and journalist Ralph Moss, the toxins work as a kind of heat therapy—"pushing the immune function to the limit of excitability." Scientists at the National Cancer Institute have discovered that a lipopolysaccharide is contained in these toxins, which appears to stimulate the immune system to produce "tumor necrosis factor" or TNF—which kills cancer.

Coley's daughter, Helen Coley Nauts, who has spent many years tabulating and publishing her father's results of nearly 1000 cases, shows that 45 percent of patients with inoperable tumors and 50 percent of those with tumors that were operable were considered cured (that is, survived for at least five years). The best results were with giant cell bone tumors and breast cancer; 79 of inoperable bone cancer patients and 87 percent of the operable patients were cured, and, among those with breast cancer, 65 percent of inoperable patients and all of the operable patients were considered cured (*Cancer Surv.*, 1989; 8: 713-23; *Prog. Clin. Biol. Rs.*, 1983; 107: 687-96).

A controlled clinical trial at NYU Medical Center in 1962 concluded that the Coley therapy "has definite oncolytic [cancer-destroying] properties and is useful in the treatment of certain types of malignant disease."

Kelley's treatment

Dr. William Kelley, an orthodontist by training, treated cancer patients for 20 years. Kelley believed that the pancreas, rather than the immune system, plays a critical role in cancer. Studies in the clinical literature lend some support to the theory that pancreatic enzymes not only serve a digestive function but also circulate in the bloodstream and kill cancer cells.

Kelley's treatment includes large doses of pancreatic enzymes, vitamin and mineral supplements, and fresh, preferably organic foods. One of 10 basic diets, some vegetarian, is prescribed to suit the patient's condition. Part of the treatment involves detoxification, assisted by coffee enemas, on the principle that caffeine administered rectally opens the bile ducts and releases accumulated toxins.

Dr. Nicholas Gonzalez, a private physician in New York, analyzed the medical records of 455 patients with a total of 26 different types of cancer treated by Kelley. Many patients, he says, were alive five, 10 or 15 years after having been diagnosed as terminal by orthodox doctors. Of the five with inoperable pancreatic cancer, four are still alive (the fifth died of Alzheimer's disease), after a median survival of 8.5 years; the conventional survival rate for this kind of cancer is three to six months.

Macrobiotics

A macrobiotic diet emphasizes whole cereal grains, beans, fresh vegetables, fruits, nuts, seeds, sea vegetables, and, occasionally, fish. Case histories of people who apparently reversed their cancers through this diet and lifestyle changes can be found in literature available from the Kushi Institute (Brookline, Massachusetts). Macrobiotics is rooted in the ancient Chinese principle of complementary yin-yang forces. According to Michio Kushi, the system's rebalancing of the body destroys some cancer cells, and causes others to change to normal ones.

Interestingly, the high-fibre, low-cholesterol, low-fat diet long advocated by a number of alternative cancer therapists shares many similarities with the diet recommendations only recently set forth in major reports of the National Academy of Sciences, the ACS, and the NCI.

Urea

The notion that human urine has anti-cancer properties has been around at least since the Second World War. However the idea has undergone a revival since the late 1950s, with the work of Dr. Evangelos D. Danopoulos, Professor of Medicine at the Medical School of Athens University, a specialist in optic oncology.

The active ingredient in urine is urea, which appears to disrupt the water system on the surface of cancer cells, which treat water differently than do normal cells, thus interfering with some of the metabolism necessary for uncontained metastasis.

In one of his many studies, Dr. Danopoulos discovered that of 46 patients with cancer in or around the eye who were treated with surgery and local urea injections, the treatment was successful in all cases. Ordinarily, conventional medicine almost never achieves a cure or remission (*Ophthal*, 1979; 179: 52-61). In another study of nine people with cancer of the mucous membrane inside the eyelid, eight out of the nine given local applications of urea were cured (*Ophthal,* 1979; 178: 198-203). Eighteen patients with liver cancer given urea survived 26.5 months, five times longer than expected (*Clinical Oncology,* 1981; 7: 281-9), as did 28 liver cancer patients, 17 with cancer that had spread (*Clinical Oncology,* 1975, I: 341-50).

Most recently, Dr. Danopoulos replaced his injected urea with a powdered variety, covered by an airtight dressing after scraping the cancerous tumor. He has achieved a cure rate as high as 96 percent (*Lancet,* 1974; i: 132).

Dr. Danopoulos discovered that creatine monohydrate has similar anti-cancer properties to urea but is broken down more slowly into creatinine. By using urea and creatine, Dr. Danopoulos found that he could keep blood levels of urea nitrogen (which fights the cancer) more consistent than with urea alone.

Hydrogen peroxide

According to the book *The UnMedical Miracle—Oxygen* by Elizabeth Baker (Delwood Communications, PO Box K, Indianola, WA 98342), hydrogen peroxide (as well as oxygen and ozone) was a widely used therapy for all sorts of illnesses in the 1920s. She claims it only fell into disuse after the advent of penicillin, when drug companies worked hard to steer doctors over to the use of pharmaceuticals.

Hydrogen peroxide (H_2O_2) is produced in the body of all higher organisms and has a key role in the body's metabolism. It is the body's first line of defense in response to microbial invasion, because it carries an extra molecule of oxygen that can be let loose to attack pathogens, which are killed by oxygen.

The theory of hydrogen peroxide therapy is that it is used to supplement the body's own supply of oxygen which, according to Baker, has fallen from 30 percent to 19 percent today (and as low as 12 percent in some cities).

The medical literature of the turn of the century is filled with successful treatment with oxygen therapy, particularly hydrogen peroxide. Numerous medical articles are beginning to advocate the use of "peroxidation" in medicine. In an article in *The Lancet* (November 12, 1988) T. G. L. Dormandy of the Department of Chemical Pathology, Whittington Hospital in London, argued that the notion of peroxidation (in connection with free radicals), has had a bad press. Far from being always evidence of damage, he says, this "self-destruct" mechanism in cells is necessary to health; failure of cells to burn themselves up and be regenerated leads to cancer.

126

Most proponents of H_2O_2 give it intravenously because it has been shown to cause venous oxygen embolism (air bubbles) when used in liquid form to irrigate surgical wounds or closed body cavities (*BMJ*, 1985; 291: 1706). Certain dilutions taken orally have also been shown to cause tumors in animals (*GANN* 1981; 72: 174-5). However, when injected at the right percentage, it quickly breaks down into oxygen and water. A recently published article from the *American Journal of Cardiology* (1993; 52: 673-5) echoed the results of numerous other studies in the 1960s, that a 0.2 percent solution of intravenous H_2O_2 can be given safely, usually with the drug heparin to avoid inflammation of a vein.

At a conference in 1989, a leading proponent of hydrogen peroxide therapy, Dr. Charles H Farr, founder of the International Bio-Oxidative Foundation in Dallas, cited many studies in the medical literature showing that hydrogen peroxide can benefit patients with many chronic degenerative diseases, and anecdotal reports of its success against candida albicans, ME and multiple sclerosis. In addition, he provided anecdotal and referenced studies of its use on cancer cells. At least one study has shown its anti-tumor effects on cells in the laboratory (*J. Exp. Med.*, 1981; 154: 1539-53).

Farr concluded (as have other studies) that when

combined with radiation therapy, hydrogen peroxide can enhance the effect and spare some normal tissue from the effects of radiation. As for its use alone, he says: "By itself it has an anti-tumor effect . . . but response is slow and changes are subtle. Responses were noted in colorectal carcinoma and malignant lymphoma." He notes, however, that there may have been problems in the studies and that larger ones, particularly double-blind studies, need to be done.

In one study, 190 patients were selected with such advanced cancer that they were considered beyond conventional treatment. In fact, less than a tenth of them were expected to survive for more than a year. After employing the hydrogen peroxide with radiation, 77 percent were alive after a year, two-thirds after two years, nearly a half after three years and one-quarter after five years. The best responders had cancer of the cervix, bladder, head or neck (*Am. J. Surgery*, 1964; 108: 621-29).

Farr finds the most successful treatment combines hydrogen peroxide therapy and high doses of vitamin C with chelation treatment, which removes the toxins of cancer from the body.

If you do opt for this approach, work only with someone highly experienced in giving such treatment to patients since the wrong infusion of oral or liquid concentration can be potentially dangerous.

Dr. Hamer's conflict theory

Unlike most other practitioners, the work of the German cancer specialist Dr. Ryke Geerd Hamer concentrates almost exclusively on the causes of cancer. Once the cause is recognized and faced, the cure will follow, he argues, as the body's own remarkable self-healing processes are freed to come into play.

Although many have testified to the success of his approach, he has been persecuted by the German authorities who have attempted to outlaw his work and stop his practicing.

In simple terms, Dr. Hamer believes that all cancers have been precipitated by a conflict. In the case of breast cancer, the shock or trauma would have occurred two to four months prior to the clinical detection of the cancer if the woman is right-handed. Cancer of the left breast would have been triggered by a perceived general conflict between a mother or child, a conflict within the family or "nest", or if the husband becomes ill or infirm. Cancer of the right breast, again in a right-handed woman, would be triggered by a conflict with humanity in general or with a partner. In left-handed women, the triggers are reversed.

Dr. Hamer has proved scientifically, his supporters say, that conflict will create a grey stress focus in the brain the size of a thumb nail. The location of the stress in the brain will determine the type of cancer that will develop.

A conflict or trauma may not seem particularly earth-shattering, certainly not to an observer, but the sense of helplessness, and of being trapped, that accompanies this stress seems to be a universal phenomenon among victims, according to Hamer.

There are also the "hanging conflicts", as Hamer defines them, which hover in a person's background, but never quite come to the surface, such as a long-held hurt.

The patient will become clear of the cancer when he or she identifies the conflict and is given the correct support on all levels—physical, mental, emotional and spiritual. No chemotherapy is needed, and Hamer regards morphine as being detrimental to the whole system. This can cause fresh conflicts and lead even to death, he believes.

Shark cartilage

Great things have been claimed for shark cartilage as a cure for cancer. Much of the existing literature about the product tells the same story. In 1975 scientists at Harvard Medical School isolated something in cartilage which prevents the growth of the tiny blood vessels which feed the tumor (angiogenesis) and which could inhibit capillary growth by 75 percent (*J. Exp. Med.*, 1975; 141: 427-39).

The following year, the same scientists discovered that cartilage contained several different proteins and that the major one strongly inhibited the activity of protein-digesting enzymes (*Sci. Am.*, 1976, 234: 58-64). A professor at Massachusetts Institute of Technology (MIT) suggested that cartilage from calves' shoulder blades would be suitable (*Science*, 1976; 193: 70-2). But, because calves' bodies contain only minute quantities of cartilage, a new source was needed, which is where sharks, whose whole internal structure is made of cartilage, came in.

Science met marketing at this point. *Sharks don't get cancer*, we were told; and "now one of man's oldest and deadliest enemies holds the key to overcoming one of modern man's most dreaded enemies." But a close look at the evidence for these claims is instructive.

Claims for shark cartilage are based mostly on *invitro* studies using chicken eggs as a model. Others are based on animal studies (*Proc. Natl. Acad. Sci*. *USA*, 1980; 77: 4331-5). Still others are based on studies on sharks which have been injected with cancerous cells to see if they would develop cancer—some did, and some didn't (*J. Pharm. Sci.*, 1977; 66: 757-8).

Angiogenesis does not cure cancer, even at very high concentrations in test tubes. MIT scientists concluded that the cartilage "does not interfere with the growth of the tumor cell population directly." Instead it simply prevents tumor growth by slowing the formation of new blood vessels (*Proc. Natl. Acad. Sci. USA,* 1980; 77: 4331-5).

Judah Foulker's work on angiogenesis is often quoted as proof that shark cartilage works. But even Prof. Foulker is clear that "in vitro assays do not accurately predict antiangiogenic efficacy in vivo"— in other words, what happens in the test tube does not necessarily reflect what happens in the body (V. T. DeVita, et al, eds., *Cancer Principles & Practice of Oncology,* Lippincott-Raven, 1997).

Books like I William Lane's *Sharks Don't Get Cancer* can be frustrating for those trying to discover the true picture. For instance, Lane quotes several small, but apparently impressive, studies supporting the efficacy of shark cartilage, but inexplicably none of these are to be found in the references at the back of the book.

While the animal studies at least used controls (so direct comparisons between those treated and those not can be made), the human studies to date amount to nothing more than case reports. For instance, Lane reports on a 1992 study in Mexico by Roscoe van Zandt in which eight women with advanced breast tumors all showed improvement after receiving shark cartilage. Similarly, of two patients in Panama with terminal cancer, one with less severe liver cancer went into remission, but the fate of the other with lung cancer which had spread to the bone and brain, was more vague.

Case studies from elsewhere in the world including unpublished data from Lane on the efficacy of anal administration tell a similar story. It is too easy to claim a 50 percent success rate when a study has only a handful of people in it. But based on these results, US TV seized on shark cartilage with enthusiasm. The well-respected program "60 Minutes" followed 27 patients in Cuba and the results, again unpublished, were even more vague: cessation of pain, improvement in appetite, attitude and quality of life. Nowhere does it say how long they stayed alive for.

Dr. Lane is not a medical doctor; his Ph.D. is in agricultural biochemistry. His company produces some of the leading shark cartilage products on the market, so he is hardly an impartial observer. Because shark cartilage is not a drug it cannot be regulated, and MIT has found that several commercially available products are without any significant potency.

Most of the supplements sold over the counter are for oral use, whereas most of the clinical studies have involved injecting the cartilage. Human studies have

been performed using both oral and anal administration. While it is clear that there may be something
in shark cartilage which does help fight cancer, there
is no evidence that the over-the-counter products in
the form of tablets, pessaries or milkshakes provide
what has now been named Cartilage-Derived
Inhibitor (CDI) in quantity or form which will deliver what it promises.

The manufacturer of one leading brand of shark
cartilage, Cartilage Technologies Inc (CTI), discontin-
ued its sponsorship of an FDA-supervised clinical
trial to evaluate shark cartilage as a treatment for
cancer. A spokesman for CTI said the company was
"unable to find meaningful scientific data to support
further investment in pursuing drug status for shark
cartilage" (*Townsend Letter for Doctors and Patients*,
April 1997: 26). CTI went on to state that it "does not
promote its product as a cancer cure and finds it difficult to understand any company that would market
a dietary supplement for the treatment of cancer,
especially when there is no basis."

Germanium
Germanium is a biological-response modifier, which
means it helps the body modify its response to
tumors. It appears to transport extra molecules of
oxygen easily inside individual cells; as cancer cells

can't metabolize oxygen, this could stop their growth or return them to normal. Its most important function may be to enhance the production of our own interferon, recognized as a powerful anti-cancer agent (*Tohoku J. Exper. Medi.*, 1985; 146: 97-104).

In a double-blind, placebo controlled study in Japan of patients with inoperable lung cancer, patients receiving germanium in addition to chemotherapy or radiation had a higher response rate and improved survival time. The treatment worked best on small cell cancers. At least 13 animal studies show evidence of anti-tumor activity (*Inter. Clin. Nutr. Review*, 1987; 7 (1): 11-20).

Nevertheless, the downside is that the inorganic form of germanium can cause kidney damage (*Renal Failure*, 1991; 13: 1-4). This damage has been caused by germanium oxide, not the organic form used in cancer patients, in all but one instance. Nevertheless, germanium can be contaminated with germanium dioxide during the process of being produced. No reliable test for purity exists.

Laetrile (amygdalin)
Found in over 1200 plants, amygdalin, also called vitamin B17, is a nitriloside found in some 1200 plants, the seeds of non-citrus fruits like apricots and peaches. When broken down by one of the enzymes

of our body, cyanide is released. Since cancer cells contain thousands of times more of this enzyme (beta-glucosidase) than normal cells, much more of the toxic cyanide is released and selectively poisonous to the cancer cells (our bodies have other enzymes which make this substance harmless to ordinary cells). Hence, in theory, amygdalin is the perfect, selective search-and-destroy substance for cancer therapy. Laetrile is the patented product of a group of doctors in San Francisco, who pioneered the use of the substance.

Studies by internationally respected research scientist Dr. Kanematsu Sugiura between 1972-7 found that amygdalin did inhibit lung metastases. Cancer researcher Dr. Ralph Moss, then a science writer at Sloan-Kettering, claims the institute covered up positive results with amygdalin (*Cancer Therapy*, Equinox Press, 1995). Another study claimed good results with breast and bone cancer patients with higher doses than had been used before (70 gm/day). Leukemia patients didn't respond (Choice, 1977; 3 (6): 8-9.

Nevertheless there have been reports of severe or fatal toxicity in children and adults, but mainly those who ingested high doses made for injection (*Pediatrics*, 1986; 78: 269-72), and usually among those self-medicating. Intravenous amygdalin appears less toxic. Avoid taking with high doses of vitamin C, which lowers the ability of normal cells to detoxify the cyanide.

NUTRITION AND VITAMINS

By far the most common and accepted of the alternative approaches (and increasingly being embraced by conventional medicine) is the use of nutrition and vitamins.

The Dries Diet

The Dries Diet, originated by Dutch nutritionist Jan Dries, is a mainly fruit diet using the bio-energetic properties of certain foods. Dries maintains that all the components of foods can be viewed as condensed light.

This view, while controversial, is not new. Bio-energetic research was started in the 1920s by the Russian scientist Alexander Gurwitsch whose work was expanded upon by Prof. Dr. Popp and his colleagues.

Dries's contribution was in recognizing the cancer-resistant qualities of some foods, especially wild berries and tropical fruits.

But perhaps the most impressive aspect of his work is the extraordinary success he has had with his many patients. He has treated well over 600 cancer patients who have incorporated his diet with other treatments with considerable success.

Vitamins

In order to see if supplementation with specific vitamins and minerals could lower cancer rates, a joint team from the US National Cancer Institute in Maryland and the Cancer Institute, Chinese Academy of Medical Sciences in Beijing, China, gave 30,000 people in Linxian County in China aged 40-69 one of four combinations of nutrients in doses roughly double the US Recommended Daily Allowance. The researchers then followed the study group over five years, to 1991.

This particular county was chosen because it has one of the world's highest rates of esophageal/gastric cancer. The inhabitants' grain-based diet is known to have a low intake of nutrients found in fruits and vegetables. The study found a 13 percent reduction in cancer deaths among the group receiving supplementation with beta carotene, vitamin E and selenium; a 10 percent reduction in mortality from all causes; and 21 percent reduction in deaths from cancer of the stomach—all striking results for so short a study period. Interestingly, the researchers also found a 38 percent reduction in mortality from cerebrovascular disease (strokes).

Although the group taking the B vitamins riboflavin and niacin did not have a statistically significant drop in overall mortality, they did show a 14 percent reduction in throat cancer and a 41 percent drop in cataracts (*J. Nat. Cancer Inst.*, Sept. 15, 1993). This study was important, because it was so carefully designed and backs up scores of similar, if smaller, studies on humans. But the message it contained is hardly new.

The Chinese study merely adds to the already weighty evidence about vitamins and cancer treatment generated from numerous similar research conducted in many countries over the past decade. Most research, like the Chinese study, has centered on the role of antioxidants in preventing or treating cancer. Antioxidants protect the body from damage caused by harmful molecules called free radicals. Besides for breathing, the body's cells use oxygen to metabolize (and literally "burn") food for its energy, and to burn away germs and toxins.

As American nutritional specialist Leo Galland puts it: "This process of combustion creates tiny bonfires in the cells, and these fires give off 'sparks' that can start fires in undesirable places, damaging cell membranes and destroying essential fatty acids." These sparks (free radicals) also are created from many other sources (ultraviolet radiation, smoke pollution, heavy metals, rancid fatty acids or over-heating of oils, such as in fast-food restaurants). Free radicals wreak havoc by destroying cell membranes, causing genetic damage, depressing immune function, hardening the arteries, disrupting hormone regulation, contributing to diabetes and other systemic disorders and, of course, causing the growth and spread of cancer.

But we're now learning that damage from free radicals can be prevented and even reversed if there are sufficient concentrations in the body of free radical scavengers, called antioxidants,—what Galland calls the body's own "fire brigade" which "snuff these sparks before they start too many fires." These include the antioxidant vitamins: A and beta-carotene, B2 (riboflavin), B3 (nicotinic acid), C and E and selenium.

Besides the Chinese study, extensive evidence supports the ability of individual antioxidants to prevent cancer. For instance, in the December 1991 issue of the *American Journal of Clinical Nutrition*, Dr. G. Block of the University of California, Berkeley, concluded that "approximately 90 epidemiologic studies have examined the role of vitamin C or vitamin C-rich foods in cancer prevention, and the vast majority have found statistically significant protective effects . . ."

But even if modern medicine is coming around to the notion that cancer can be prevented by diet and nutrients, it is less willing to use these tools to fight cancer that is already there. Most oncologists aren't aware of (or don't accept) the massive research during the past decade on the treatment of cancer using nutritional supplements. The Bristol Cancer Help Centre—which offers complementary and alternative cancer treatments—has been compiled a database of 3000 research studies in this area. This research is not the work of fringe organizations, but of prestigious scientists and laboratories published in mainstream medical journals.

Much of the data concerns work on cells or animals and some of the work on people is preliminary. Nevertheless, the existence of this copious research is all the more reason to wonder why the medical profession continues to treat the use of nutritional therapy for cancer as anything other than a feel-good adjunct to the "real" treatment—radiation, chemotherapy or surgery—when that treatment hasn't made any headway in terms of improving survival statistics since the time of our grandparents (*New Eng. J. Med.*; 1986; 314: 1226-32).

Vitamin A/beta carotene

Fat-soluble vitamin A, vital to eye and retina function (whence its name retinol is derived), protects the mucous membranes of the mouth, nose, throat and lungs from damage, and as an immune system enhancer, reduces risk of infection and cancer. Researchers suggest that retinol may reduce cancer risk because of its role in maintaining cell integrity and because certain retinoids have been shown to stop the growth of chemically induced tumors in laboratory animals.

These days, most scientists agree that the benefits have more to do with beta carotene, which the body metabolizes into vitamin A, making only what it needs. While you can overdose on fat-soluble vitamin A, found in liver and fish, large doses of water-soluble beta carotene, found in carrots and broccoli, are non-toxic and constitute an extremely potent source of antioxidants.

Almost every study of nutrition and cancer shows a relationship between low levels of vitamin A and cancer, including the otherwise conservatively interpreted results of the Harvard's Nurses' Health study of 90,000 women with breast cancer (*New England Journal of Medicine*, July 22, 1993).

Work in the laboratory on cell lines and animals has shown that vitamin A/beta carotene also has a direct toxic effect upon cancer cells. Researchers at Harvard School of Dental Medicine found that beta carotene or vitamin E quickly altered and slowed proliferation of in vitro breast, oral, lung and skin human tumor cell lines (*J. Oral. Maxillofac. Surg.;* Apr. 1992).

Of the human studies that are available, a number have showed that beta carotene and vitamin A can help reverse pre-cancerous lesions. One Canadian study showed that tobacco chewers from Kerala, India, given vitamin A for six months, oral pre-cancerous lesions completely disappeared in slightly more than half and virtually all experienced a reduction in abnormal cells. Beta carotene produced similar results. Vitamin A also stopped the formation of new lesions (*Am. J. Clin. Nutr.,* Jan. 1991).

According to American health writer Gary Null (*Healing Your Body Naturally*, Four Walls Eight Windows, 1992) studies done at the Sloan-Kettering Institute in Manhattan have found that a vitamin A derivative caused a remission in 80 percent of subjects with leukemia—with far greater results than among those receiving chemotherapy as well.

However, several recent studies, including one conducted in Helsinki, Finland (*NEJM,* 14 April, 1994), found that smokers who take beta-carotene increase their risks of developing the disease. The reasons for this are not clear. The answer may lie in the general effect smoking has on nutrients. For example, it is known that smoking greatly increases an individual's vitamin C requirements. Or it may be something peculiar to the study group, many of whom had been smoking for 36 years, and 18 percent of whom had worked in mines and quarries, or with insulation that had particles known to cause cancer.

During the five- to eight-year trial period, 876 new cases of lung cancer were reported among the participants, with little difference between the groups. There was an 18 percent higher incidence among the beta carotene group (*NEJM*, 14 April, 1994).

It may be that beta carotene supplements could be suppressing other cancer fighters in the body, especially in someone with a low nutritional status. A better source of beta carotene may be from fruit and vegetables.

This theory has been given some weight by American nutritionist Dr. Alan Gaby. He looked at two volunteers who took 25 mg of beta carotene and 25 mg of the carotenoid canthaxanthin.

When the supplements were taken together, the blood concentration of canthaxanthin fell by 38 percent, suggesting that beta carotene inhibits canthaxanthin (*Townsend Letter for Doctors*, December 1995).

Vitamin C

Perhaps more research has been performed on vitamin C than on any other nutrient, largely due to the interest of twice Nobel Prize laureate research scientist Linus Pauling.

Thirty years ago, Scottish surgeon Dr. Ewan Cameron postulated that any substance which strengthened the intercellular cement binding cells together would probably help to resist invasion by malignant tumor cells. Vitamin C prompts cells to produce higher levels of hyaluronidase inhibitor, which prevents the hyaluronidase produced by cancer cells from breaking down this cement between cells. Vitamin C also helps strengthen the cement itself by helping to synthesize collagen (Ross Pelton and Lee Overholder, *Alternatives in Cancer Therapy*, Fireside, 1994). We also know that vitamin C stimulates natural killer (NK) cell activity.

In addition to being a potent antioxidant, vitamin C enhances antiviral and anti-bacterial immune function. Most studies of stomach and esophageal cancers have shown that the diets of the adult patients are low in vitamin C-rich foods (*Epidemiology*, 1991; 2: 325-57). The Chinese trial showed no evidence of reduced cancer among the group given vitamin C alone; however, it may be that the doses—only twice the US Recommended Daily

Allowance—were too low, far lower than doses recommended by Pauling and others for therapeutic purposes.

A Canadian study, which performed a combined analysis of data from 12 studies of diet and breast cancer, predicted that dietary changes including vitamin C could prevent about a fifth of all breast cancers (*J. Natl. Cancer Inst.*; April 4, 1990).

At present we really don't understand how vitamin C works, but some of the studies suggest that something in its chemistry, rather than its properties as a vitamin, inhibit a variety of cancers—breast, liver and leukemias. In the case of estrogen-dependent breast cancer, vitamin C has the ability to lower the concentration of toxic hormonal substances produced by estrogens.

The Linus Pauling Institute in California found vitamin C had a similar inhibiting factor on breast cancer tumors implanted in mice (*Am. J. Clin. Nutr.*, Dec. 1991), and the University of Texas in Galveston demonstrated vitamin C's ability to decrease estrogen-induced tumor growth in hamster kidneys by half (Am J Clin Nutr, Dec 1991).

The US National Cancer Institute has been taking a hard look at the effects of vitamin C on the body, particularly its alleged ability to treat cancer. Although two controlled clinical trials sponsored by the cancer institute have concluded the vitamin was ineffective in advanced cases of cancer, the institute found numerous epidemiological studies that were more optimistic. Of 46 studies, 33 showed evidence of statistically significant treatment of cancers of the mouth, esophagus, stomach, pancreas, breast, anus, colon and cervix.

After teaming up with Pauling, Dr. Cameron gave vitamin C to 100 Scottish cancer patients, who'd been considered beyond treatment. The vitamin C patients survived four times as long (210 days) as 1000 similar patients not given the vitamin (*Proc. Natl. Aca. Sci.*, 1976; 73: 3685-9). Another study also showed that the vitamin C group lived nearly a year more than those not receiving it, but many lived on for years, while all those not receiving the supplement eventually died (*Proc. Natl. Acad. Sci.*, 1978; 75: 4538-42). A later study with lung cancer patients had similar results (*J. Int. Acad. Prev. Med.*, 1979; 6: 21-7).

Then in 1990, Pauling and Canadian biochemist and psychiatrist Dr. Abram Hoffer published a study examining the survival of cancer patients on a nutritional program. Those who did not use vitamins survived for an average of only 5.7 months. Of those taking daily supplements, which included beta-carotene and 10 grams of vitamin C, 80 percent lived 16 times as long as the control patients, and many were still alive at the time the paper was written. The best responders were women with breast, ovarian and fallopian-tube cancers (*J. Ortho. Med.,* 1990; 5: 143-54).

Vitamin E

Vitamin E has a particular antioxidant role on cell membranes, at times working in tandem with vitamin C, and interacting with vitamin A, the B-complex vitamins and selenium. It prevents toxic interaction with fats and oxygen in cells and so plays a vital role in maintaining the cell's integrity and use of oxygen. As an immune system enhancer, vitamin E especially protects against lung damage from pollution.

In a Boston animal study, vitamin E prevented oral tumor formation in hamsters by galvanizing the immune system to destroy developing tumor cells (*J. Oral. Pathol. Med.,* Feb. 1990). The largest controlled human study in Italy to date has shown that the risk of stomach cancer was more closely linked to low intake of vitamin E than any other nutrient (*Int. J. Cancer,* 45: 896-901, 1990), and a national study of over 1000 American patients showed that vitamin E supplements reduced the risk of oral cancer by half (*Am. J. Epidemiol.,* 1992; 135: 1083-92,). As for treatment, of 43 patients at the Anderson Cancer Center in Houston, Texas, with precancerous oral lesions treated with vitamin E, nearly half improved and a fifth showed evidence of cell improvement after six months (*J. Natl. Cancer Inst., Jan.* 6, 1993).

The Finnish study (mentioned earlier) which found increased lung cancer among smokers taking beta carotene, also found no reduction in the cancer among those taking vitamin E supplements.

Selenium

Selenium, whose best source is seafood, works in partnership with vitamin E to protect against cancer and to prevent cell membrane damage. This mineral detoxifies heavy metals, protects against environmental and chemical sensitivities, and enhances the body's antibacterial and antiviral defenses. A variety of animal and human studies point to its ability to inhibit colon, cervical, breast and liver cancers.

A study in Finland, for instance, found that blood levels of selenium were significantly lower in men who went on to develop stomach cancer (*J. Natl. Cancer Insti.,* 1990; 82: 864-868). In American Health Foundation research, selenium inhibited colon and breast cancer in rats (*Cancer Res.,* May 1 and Oct 15, 1992). And research at Nehru University, New Delhi, India, found that administering selenium in drinking water reduced cervical cancer incidence by half in mice (*Oncology;* 1992; 49: 237-40).

Essential Fatty Acids

In all the attention focused on antioxidants, the role of essential fatty acids in protecting and treating cancer and maintaining a healthy immune system tends to get overlooked.

Fats are broadly divided into saturated and polyunsaturated. There are two kinds of EFAs—called "essential" because the body needs them but cannot manufacture them itself: omega-6 linoleic acid and gamma-linolenic acid (present in evening primrose oil), and the omega-3 alpha linolenic acid family (found in fish and linseed oils). Broadly speaking, these acids get metabolized into hormone-like substances called prostaglandins, which regulate the activity of the white blood cells in the immune system.

We're not sure how EFAs kill tumor cells but it may involve the ability of fatty acids to bind to protein and so prevent the toxic action of tumor cells (*Nutrition*, Sept.-Oct., 1992).

Perhaps most important of all are those studies that examine all the anti-oxidants working in tandem. The Chinese study, mentioned earlier, where only the group with the highest number of antioxidants had improved cancer survival, suggests that antioxidant nutrients may rely on an interaction with each other to produce the best results.

Although much of the laboratory and clinical evidence is impressive, some of the studies that have been done to treat human cancer patients with nutrients have been small or inconclusive. In a companion trial done in the same province of China on 3000 people with esophageal cancer, there was no significant survival difference between the group given 26 vitamins and those given a placebo. Again, this may be because treatment requires megadoses, and the study group was only receiving two or three times the RDA. While epidemiologic evidence consistently shows that people eating lots of fresh fruit and vegetables reduce their risks of cancer by as much as a half (*Epidemiology*, 1991; 2: 325-57), we still have much to learn about the dosage in treating people once they have the disease.

Green vegetables

Apart from the nutrients discussed above, there may be other elements in food which can protect against cancer. Researchers from John Hopkins University in Baltimore, found that broccoli, brussel sprouts, cauliflower, cress and other vegetables of the cruciferae family all contain a chemical called sulforaphane, which apparently has anti-cancer properties.

OTHER ALTERNATIVES

Homeopathy

Homeopaths claim some success with tailoring therapies for individuals to control symptoms or the response to more aggressive treatments (*Br. Hom. J.,* 1993; 82: 179-85), and with leukemia (*Br. Hom. J.,* 1986; 75 (2): 96-101). Furthermore, in some experimental trials, it has been shown that in cancer cells, the ionic balance, (which regulates cell differentiation), is disturbed.

Homeopaths have sought to re-establish the ionic equilibrium by administering biochemical salts in small quantities. In laboratory experiments, Kali phos (30x), Calc phos (30x) and Ferrum phos (30x) have all shown anti-tumor effects. In 20 women with cervical cancer, treated with Kali mur, Ferrum phos, Calc phos and Silicea, three had a remarkable regression of their cancer and seven, a slight regression (*Br. Hom. J.,* 1983; 72: 99-103). Other studies have shown that a proprietary homeopathic extract Ukrain (derived from Chelidonium) has a marked destructive effect on tumor cell lines in the laboratory (*J. Chemotherapy,* 1996; 8: 144-6).

Herbs

Herbs have a long history—and much scientific evidence—demonstrating their anti-cancer effects.

One reason the Japanese have the highest tobacco smoking rate but the lowest lung cancer rate could be green tea. The tea contains epigallocatechin gallate, theophylline, tannic acid and other polyphenols, which have been shown to inhibit cancer growth (*Jpn. J. Cancer Res.*, 1989, 80: 503-5).

In 1975, the Journal of the US National Cancer Institute reported that a number of derivatives of marijuana (*Cannabis sativa*) were clearly shown to retard both the growth of lung cancer and spleen enlargement in mice with leukemia. Survival time was lengthened by up to 36 percent (*J. Nat. Cancer Inst.*, 1975, 55: 597-602).

Certain parts of sorrel rhubarb (*Rheum palmatum*) and Indian rhubarb (*Rheum rhaponticum*) contain rhein, catechin and aloe emodin, which have been shown to have anti-tumor activity (*J. Nat. Cancer Inst.*, 1952, 13: 139-155).

Investigators at the US University of Virginia, Charlottesville, reported that aloe emodin, which is also present in Alder Buckthorn bark and seeds (*Rhamnus frangula*), showed "significant anti-leukemic activity in mice" (*Lloydia,* 1976, 39: 223-4).

Burdock root (*Arctium lappa*), present in both the herbal combinations used in Hoxsey's herbs (see later) and Essiac, has confirmed anti-tumor properties (*Acta. Phys. Chem.,* 1964, 10: 91-3; Tumori, 1966, 52: 173).

Echinacea has evidence of indirect cancer-fighting activity because of its long-recognized ability to boost the immune system. (Z)-1,8-pentadecadiene, a fat-soluble component of *E angustifolia* and *E pallida*, has been shown in the laboratory to have significant cancer-cell killing ability (*J. Med. Chem.*, 1972; 15: 619-23).

In 1984, Japanese investigators at Kawasaki Medical School in Hondo Island isolated an anti-mutation factor in burdock root, which turned out to be resistant to protein-digesting enzymes and heat. They named it the "burdock factor", which has been shown to render virtually innocuous a wide range of substances known to cause carcinogenic mutation (*Mutat. Res.*, 1984, 129: 25-31). One important component of burdock is benzaldehyde, also present in Laetrile, or amygdalin, found primarily in the kernels of plums, apricots, peaches and bitter almonds.

In 1985 Dr. M. Kochi and colleagues treated 65 inoperable cancer patients with benzaldehyde, and reported an overall response rate of 55 percent, with seven patients achieving complete response, 29 achieving partial response, and 24, no further progression of disease (*Cancer Treat. Rep.*, 1985, 69: 533-7). These results have been repeated in another study, which achieved an overall response rate of 58.3 percent (*Brit. J. Cancer*, 1990, 62: 436-9). In both studies the conclusion was that they produced significant anti-cancer effects without toxicity. A Norwegian trial found that benzaldehyde changed malignant cells back to normal (*Anticancer Res.*, 1991; 11: 1077-81).

The herb *Astragalus oxyphysus* contains the alkaloid swainsonine, which has been shown to help the spleen stop the spread of cancer to other areas of the body. Animal research conducted at the US Howard University Cancer Centre demonstrates that this herb can stop the spread of melanoma (*Cancer Res.*, 1988, 48: 1410-5).

Within a day of being added to the drinking water of mice, it had inactivated more than 80 percent of tumors in their lungs. This was likely due to enhanced activation of the natural killer cell function. Swainsonine has also been shown to slow the rate of growth of human melanoma cells (*Cancer Res.*, 1990, 50: 1867-72).

The Journal of the National Cancer Institute has concluded that swainsonine causes anti-cancer activity on any sort of tumor (*J. Nat. Cancer Inst.*, 1989, 81: 1024-8).

Iscador therapy

Iscador is the proprietary name (by Weleda) of an extract containing European mistletoe, a semi-parasitic plant which was favored as a cancer treatment by Rudolf Steiner in the 1920s. It's often used to shrink a tumor before and after surgery and radiotherapy, although it has been used on its own, by injection, to treat patients with cervical, ovarian, breast, stomach, lung and colon cancer.

Iscador

Mistletoe contains several chemicals which seem to effectively fight cancer while boosting the immune system; an enzyme appears to inhibit the reproduction of cells. But unlike chemotherapy, which kills cells wholesale, good and bad, mistletoe stimulates killer white blood cells which selectively terminate cancer cells alone.

In one trial at the Lucas Clinic Laboratory of Immunology in Arlesheim, Switzerland, a single injection of Iscador given to 20 breast cancer patients were found to have significant increases in both killer cell immune responses and cell-inhibiting effect (*Oncology*, 1986: 43 (suppl 1): 51-6).

Of 25 women with primary cancer of the ovary given Iscador after surgery, all the women with stage I and II disease, and a quarter of those with stage III (none in stage IV) were alive after five years. These were compared with similar ovarian cancer patients treated with Cytoval, another cancer treatment. Even though the Iscador patients had a worse prognosis (20 of the women were in the advanced stages of III and IV), those given mistletoe lived an average of three times as long (16.2 months) as those given Cytoval (*Onkologie*, 1979; 2 (1): 28-36). It should be noted that Iscador is potentially toxic with serious side effects when too much is taken. Never attempt to make your own kitchen extract, since both leaves and berries can be poisonous.

Hoxsey's herbs

Harry Hoxsey, an ex-coalminer, used a herbal cancer remedy reportedly handed down through his family since 1840, when his great-grandfather devised the formula after watching a cancerous horse cure itself by grazing on medicinal herbs.

The basic formula, taken internally or externally, uses nine herbs, including licorice, red clover, cascara, burdock root and stillingia root. A dietary regime, vitamins and immune stimulation are part of the Hoxsey therapy as practiced today.

By 1955, Hoxsey's Dallas clinic, with over 12,000 patients, was the world's largest privately-owned cancer treatment facility. Hoxsey was frequently arrested for practicing without a license. In 1960, his clinics were banned in the US. He died in 1974. Today his former chief nurse continues the therapy at the Bio-Medical Center in Tijuana, Mexico.

The AMA labeled Hoxsey a dangerous quack, but refused to investigate the Hoxsey medicines or to evaluate their efficacy. Yet two federal courts upheld the "therapeutic value" of Hoxsey's internal tonic, and a 1953 federal report to Congress confirmed Hoxsey's charges of a "conspiracy" by the AMA, NCI, and FDA to "suppress" an impartial assessment of his methods. The AMA later admitted that Hoxsey's external medication had merit. Barberry Root, prickly ash and stillingia have shown anti-tumor activities, by only in animal tests (Pelton and Overholser, *Alternatives in Cancer Therapy*, Fireside, 1994).

Chinese remedies

In Chinese medicine, the herb *Epimediia glycoside icariine* (ICA) has been shown to boost the body's defenses by increasing NK cell and lymphokine-activated killer cell (LAK) activity and to stimulate the production of TNF in both tumor patients and healthy people (*Arzneimittel-Forschung*, 1995; 45: 910-3).

Another herb, *Shosaiko-to* (TJ-9), has been shown in the laboratory to have anti-tumor effects and to prevent liver cancer in patients with cirrhosis (Cancer, 1995; 76: 743-9). *Ninjin Yoh eito* extract granules have been demonstrated to improve the quality of life of lung cancer patients after chemotherapy (*Ther. Res.*, 1994; 15: 487-500).

Other Chinese herbs with some clinical success are *Actinidia, Baohuoside-1, Mylabris, Liu Wei Di Huang* or *Jin Gui Shen Qi* and *Buzhong Yiqi* (Moss, *Cancer Therapy*, Equinox Press, 1995).

TRUE STORIES OF SURVIVORS

Near to home

Our first case study couldn't be closer to home. It concerns the now 81-year-old mother of *What Doctors Don't Tell You* publisher Bryan Hubbard and the work and methods of Dr. Patrick Kingsley, a doctor based in Leicestershire, England.

The story began on a Sunday in March, 1993, when Bryan's father told him in confidence that his mother was to see the local doctor the following day because lumps had developed on one of her breasts. The following evening his father phoned with the shattering news that the lumps were, indeed, malignant, but they were so advanced that it was too late to perform chemotherapy or any other intervention. The doctor prescribed tamoxifen and morphine as a powerful painkiller.

It appears Bryan's mother had been secretly nursing the lumps for 18 months and had been dressing what had become open ulcerated sores.

So powerful was the morphine that his mother collapsed in the street and again at home. Bryan spoke to the doctor who believed this was a direct result of the cancer. The doctor tried to prepare the family for death, which he estimated would be within three months.

It was obvious to Bryan that the morphine, and not the cancer, was causing his mother to collapse. He suggested she come off the morphine and, to her credit, she agreed. The next challenge was greater. Fortunately, Bryan was well aware of the good work of Dr. Patrick Kingsley, particularly in treating MS sufferers. But could he help people with terminal cancer?

So confident was Dr. Kingsley that the family were able to convey that assurance back to Bryan's mother who, from the outset, was to believe implicitly that Dr. Kingsley could and would cure her. Nothing would make her waiver from that view, even though Dr. Kingsley's treatment must have been far removed from anything she had experienced before.

His first concern was her diet. After a blood test, he immediately put her on a strict exclusion diet which cut out many of the foods and drink—dairy products, wheat and the like—that formed the staple of her daily regimen. The treatment must have seemed equally as bizarre. Dr. Kingsley believes cancer can be treated with very large dosages of vitamin C and other antioxidants. This is aided by intravenous doses of hydrogen peroxide; oxygen is lethal when introduced directly into the blood stream, but apparently safe when administered in this method.

The diet is also vital in the treatment. Patrick maintains that many people have allergic reactions to many everyday foods which can trigger disease and also inhibit the body's natural defenses.

For the first month or so, Bryan's mother would make trips to Dr. Kingsley's surgery in a small village called Osgathorpe twice a week for her intravenous treatment.

She immediately started to look better, presumably a combination of the drugs and the restriction on the foods that were apparently giving her an allergic reaction. But was she really going to be cured?

It is a question on which Dr. Kingsley would never be drawn. The cancer might recede (and so presumably could return if she returned to her "poisonous" diet) but a patient was never cured as such, or so it appeared.

Cure or no, Bryan's mother was making great strides. Within three months, her visits were down to one a week, the health visitor was calling just once a week—instead of every day—to dress her wounds, and she was starting to take the vitamins in powder form to complement the intravenous treatments.

The lumps soon disappeared, the sores —save one

—completely healed, and she finished by visiting Patrick just once every six weeks. The local doctor who had issued the death sentence asked to see her breast. It was a look to treasure, according to Bryan's mother afterwards. To that doctor, it was a recovery of a sort he had never seen before.

Although women are urged to seek help at the first sign of a lump, in Bryan's mother's case, it was lucky she waited so long. Most likely, it was only because medicine considered her a lost cause that she agreed to go along with Dr. Kingsley's unconventional treatment.

In a sense Mrs. Hubbard is very rare—one of the few patients who has had nutritional treatment with no orthodox intervention—none of the cutting, burning or poisoning that might have weakened her system further. Equally significant may have been unswerving belief and trust in her doctor. This had a lot to do with Dr. Kingsley's approach when she first saw him, his refusal to be discouraged by cancer or to betray any doubt. His confidence gave her hope, and hope is saving her life.

Another essential factor was his steadfast refusal to characterize the likely path of her illness—to make a judgement about "how long" the illness would linger or how long she would live. Very few doctors have the humility to realize that no scientist, no matter how learned, can predict how a given patient will respond to the challenge of illness and healing, or say with certainty who will live and who will die.

A remarkable response

A patient of homeopath, acupuncturist and expert in nutritional and herbal medicine, George Lewith (who also works at the University of Southampton and in London), visited him in February 1996 after a clear diagnosis of pancreatic cancer, one of the most deadly.

He had gone to his GP just before Christmas 1995 with weight loss and tiredness. On examination, he was shown to have a mass, probably a tumor, in his upper abdomen and a provisional diagnosis of cancer was made. Ultrasound scans suggested both liver and peritoneal secondaries, and this was confirmed through an exploratory operation when biopsies were taken and the exact nature of the tumor defined as an adenocarcinoma.

The prognosis for this particular condition is poor. Patients would usually be expected to continue to lose weight and continue to see local tumor growth in association with symptoms such as nausea and abdominal pain. The tumor might also start to obstruct the free flow of fecal material through the bowels.

Because of the levels of secondary growth, surgery

was impractical and, after some discussion with his GP and oncologist, the patient decided that he did not wish to undergo treatment either with anti-cancer drugs or with radiotherapy, as these would be very likely to create serious adverse reactions, and the evidence for their effectiveness in this kind of cancer is limited.

He went to see Lewith to discuss the using of complementary medical techniques to manage his problem. Lewith adopted a four-pronged attack. The first was to provide advice on diet. The patient was started on a regime high in wholefoods and fresh organic food and low in animal fats and processed foods. He also started high doses of nutritional supplements, specifically vitamin C, zinc, selenium and vitamin B complex.

Simultaneously, a number of homeopathic mixtures were provided, some taken orally and some by injection. The oral medications were in the form of homeopathic complexes targeted largely at the liver and pancreas as well as homeopathic doses of shark's cartilage. The injectable preparation, Iscador, was also used, the strength of which was progressively increased until a maintenance dose was ascertained based on the clinical response after three months.

The patient was also placed on a high dose of fish-oil supplements.

Much to the surprise of the patient's GP, his clinical oncologist—and his homeopath—he has continued to improve over the last eight months and has put on the best part of 14 lbs. It appears, on examination, that his tumor has diminished substantially. After an original diagnosis of three to six months to live, to all intents and purposes, he is now clinically well.

5

Advice

WHAT DO YOU DO
IF YOU'VE GOT CANCER?

● If you plan to seek solutions through conventional medicine, find the most experienced surgeon who will treat you as an equal partner in any treatment decisions.

● Insist on the most conservative surgery possible; if over 60 with breast cancer, explore the possibility of taking a drug like tamoxifen alone.

● If you do take tamoxifen, make sure to have periodic tests on your eyes, liver and womb (endometrium), and take any drug or radiation therapies for the shortest possible time. Remember, if you haven't gone through menopause yet, no studies have proved that tamoxifen will work for you.

● Don't hesitate to take the best from conventional and alternative therapies and use them together. Contact an organization like the Bristol Cancer Help

Centre, or the American International Hospital and clinic, which offer a variety of approaches to cancer (see p. 179 for details).

The Bristol Cancer Help Centre employs a holistic approach encompassing diet, exercise, meditation, relaxation, visualization, and even psychology—in order to help you to change the lifestyle that has made you ill.

- Read books by Bernie Siegel and Louise Hay. Dr. Siegel is a surgeon who nevertheless believes (as do an increasing number of immunologists) that your mind can help your body to heal. He encourages his patients to use complementary therapies like visualization and diet, whether or not they use chemotherapy and surgery. Louise Hay beat cancer with this body/mind approach.
- Don't be a "good" patient. Many studies have demonstrated that patients who speak up for their rights and refuse to accept gloomy prognoses live longer than those who unthinkingly follow doctors' orders. Above all, don't accept a death sentence.

A recipe for nutritional cancer treatment

If you have cancer and would like to use a nutritional approach, either instead of or in tandem with conventional approaches:

- Don't embark on this form of treatment unless you

firmly believe that it will work for you. Any form of treatment—conventional or alternative—works best in people who believe in it.

• Find a practitioner who is highly experienced and successful in using dietary manipulation and supplements in cancer treatment, alone or in combination with other approaches. Find out the survival rate of his patients.

• Stop smoking and drinking alcohol and caffeine.

• Eat food and drink water which is as pure and chemically unadulterated as possible. Eat whole foods, preferably organic, especially whole grains, pulses, vegetables and fruits. Eat white meat only (fish, chicken, turkey).

• Use the highest quality unprocessed cold-pressed oils such as extra virgin olive oil for frying, and safflower and sunflower for salads. Avoid margarine; use a little butter if you must.

• Take high doses of nutritional supplements as prescribed for your individual requirements.

General guidelines for treating or preventing cancer:
Vitamin A 10,000 IU, Beta Carotene 25,000 IU, Vitamin B complex 50-100 mg, Vitamin C 3-10 g, Vitamin E 600-800 mcg, Selenium 100-200 mcg, Essential Fatty Acids (Omega-3)—1-2 Fish Oil or flax capsules or one tbs. of flax oil per day.

• Those patients who most successfully fight cancer combine a dietary and supplement program with the use of cancer-fighting substances—rather than simply seeking out a "magic bullet" which is going to kill their cancer.

In one study of patients with pancreatic cancer, which usually has a survival time of about four months, those receiving a mix of treatments—vitamins A and E, enzyme therapy, hyperthermia, tamoxifen, mistletoe, thymus extract and other substances to boost the immune system—trebled the usual survival rate, and reported improved quality of life, with a gain of appetite and weight, and pain relief (*Erfahrungsheilkunde*, 1996; 45: 64-72).

• Follow a high-fibre, low-fat, low-protein diet, rich in dark green, leafy and yellow vegetables (*Int. J. Cancer*, 1990; 45: 899-901). Lowering fat may enhance the function of your immune system and increase NK cell activity which can help reduce the spread of the disease (*Am. J. Clin. Nutr.*, 1989; 50: 861-7).

• Don't fry foods and do limit eggs, as well as hydrogenated fats and smoked, salt-cured or pickled foods, sugar and too much salt. Vegetarian diets appear to be protective, as do soy products. The Kelley dietary program, which has 10 types of individually tailored diets, also has some evidence of success (*What Doctors Don't Tell You*, vol 7, no 3).

• Some therapists recommend thymus extract to boost the immune system. Omega-3 and -6 fatty acids have been shown to kill cancer. As for minerals, too much calcium has been related to cancer (*Br. Med. J.*, 1989; 298: 1468-9) as have high levels of iron (*N. Engl. J. Medi.*, 1988; 319: 1047-52), although at appropriate levels, both are protective. Selenium, magnesium, iodine and zinc all fight cancer. Germanium, another mineral, appears to enhance the production of our body's own interferon (*Tohoku J. Exper. Med.*, 1985; 146: 97-104).

• Drink hard, rather than soft water (*J. Orthomol . Med.*, 1989; 4 (2): 59-69) and avoid chlorine and fluoride, which have both been implicated in cancer.

• Consider a number of substances which act as cancer inhibitors, even if on their own they don't actually cure. These can help in conjunction with more potent anti-cancer agents. These include:

Melatonin

Melatonin can amplify the anti-tumor effect of a variety of substances. In one study of patients with spreading tumors untreatable by conventional means, nearly half the patients given melatonin and interleukin-2—which helps the immune system fight cancer—were alive a year later, compared to only eight out of 48 of those given support alone (*Supp.*

Care Cancer, May 1995). Similar results have been achieved in patients with brain tumors given melatonin alone (*Cancer*, 1994; 73: 699-701), as well as those with cancer of the stomach (*Tumori*, December 31, 1993) and lung (Oncology, 1992; 49 (5): 336-9).

Bovine cartilage

The research on bovine cartilage appears superior to that of shark cartilage (which also provides excessive amounts of calcium). In one study, of 31 terminal cancer patients, 35 percent showed a complete response with probable or possible cures (*J. Biol. Response Modifiers*, 1985; 4: 583).

Mind-body therapies

Engage in deep relaxation, meditation, visualization, regular exercise and support groups.

The natural way to prevent prostate cancer

In the US, the National Academy of Sciences estimates that 40 percent of men's cancers, especially prostate cancer, are affected by nutrition.

• A low-fat, high fibre, high-complex carbohydrate diet, (and avoiding alcohol) helps to reduce the risk of prostate cancer.

• Fat intake, more often than any other dietary factor, has repeatedly been found to be related to the risk of cancer, and some studies suggest that the amount of saturated fat in your diet may be particularly important. A study which included five ethnic groups—Japanese, Caucasian, Chinese, Filipino, and Hawaiian —showed that reducing fat intake reduced the risk of prostate cancer (*Am. J. Nut.*, 1991; 53: 31 and 54: 1093-100).

● Eat soy products. In Japan and some other Asian countries, death from prostate cancer is low (Int J Cancer 1982; 29: 611-616) because their diet is not only low in fat but also contains a high content of soy products, a rich source of isoflavanoids which inhibit the growth of prostate cancer (*The Lancet* 1993; 342: 1209-10).

● Increase your fibre intake. A study of Seventh-Day Adventist men—who eat a lot of beans, lentils, peas and some dried fruits—showed that the more fibre a person consumes (especially lignin and the water-insoluble fibers, such as cellulose), the greater was the binding to estrogen and testosterone, thus reducing the amount of these hormones in the body and possibly reducing the risk of prostate cancer (Cancer, 1989; 64: 589-604; and *Am. J. Clin. Nut.*, 1990; 51: 365-70).

● Avoid estrogen in processed food. A review in the *Journal of Endocrinology* (1993; 136: 357-60) suggests that exposure at birth to estrogenic chemicals in foods such as cows' milk may be connected to a decline in sperm counts and a doubling in the rate of testicular cancer among men in Western countries.

● Eat zinc-rich foods and consider zinc supplements. A healthy prostate contains higher levels of zinc than any other organ, because it's required for producing male hormones. Zinc protects us from the toxic effects of the metal cadmium, which has been shown to stimulate the growth of the prostate in low concentrations. High-level exposure to cadmium is associated with an increased risk of prostate and lung cancer (*Am. J. Epidemiol.*, 1989; 129: 112-24). Compared with other groups, men with the most malignant form of prostate cancer have the highest cadmium levels and the lowest zinc levels. Pilot studies have shown that zinc supplements can successfully reduce an enlarged prostate and treat the associated symptoms. It's therefore suggested that a daily 15 mg dose forms part of of your diet, no matter what other treatment plan you're on.

● Make sure you have enough essential fatty acids, particularly omega-6 variety, found in evening primrose oil. Linoleic acid has been shown to reduce the risk of cancer cells forming within the prostate (*Nutr. Cancer* 1987; 9: 123-28).

● Consider taking botanical extracts of pollen and saw palmetto. Both have been shown in studies to reduce symptoms of benign prostate enlargement and shrink prostate size.

TWO HOLISTIC APPROACHES

Dr. PATRICK KINGSLEY

The mainstay of Dr. Patrick Kingsley's (see page 159) treatment is a combination of high-dose, intravenous vitamin C and intravenous oxygen therapy of hydrogen peroxide.

Dr. Kingsley advises patients to avoid junk food, refined carbohydrates, tea, coffee, milk and dairy products, some grains, particularly wheat, and yeasts.

Instead they should consume soya products and fresh fruits and vegetables, particularly the cruciferous variety (broccoli, cauliflower), which have proven anti-oxidant effects. Changes to diet should be introduced slowly, to minimize stress.

They are also advised to take at least 10 g. of powdered vitamin C per day (magnesium ascorbate, to maximize gut tolerance), a good antioxidant mixture, and 7-10 g. of the herb echinacea per day (which stimulates the immune system).

He also believes that coffee enemas are useful, because they stimulate the liver and large intestine into excreting toxic elements from the body. Colonics Too

Dr. Kingsley cites anecdotal evidence of his success. Recently at a local cancer self-help group, of 36 of his patients, 24, or two-thirds, said that they were rid of the cancer or continually improving. Four patients had reached a plateau, two patients were deteriorating and six not improving. Dr. Kingsley says that this percentage outcome is fairly typical.

NICHOLAS GONZALEZ

Nicholas Gonzalez is a New York immunologist who follows many of orthodontist Dr. William Kelley's theories in treating advanced cancer patients—principally, that it is the pancreas, rather than the immune system, which is critical in cancer control (see p 134).

He advises patients to adopt an individualized, fresh, organic diet (one of 10, from vegetarian to high meat, depending on your cancer and constitution).

His patients are put on high-dose supplements and pancreatic enzymes which are believed to attack and liquify tumors. They are given digestive aids and concentrates of raw beef organs and glands. They also undergo detoxification, particularly with coffee enemas.

An extensive study of 50 patients treated by Kelley with terminal or extremely poor prognosis shows apparently impressive results. All are alive 10 years after the study. Of five patients with pancreatic cancer, four are still alive (the fifth died of Alzheimer's disease) after 10 years. Their survival with conventional treatment would be three to five months.

The Sun

With controversy surrounding the use of sunscreens, there are alternative ways of avoiding burning which should be used in combination with careful, controlled exposure.

Vitamin A supplements and their close cousins, the carotenoids, may reduce the likelihood of burning. Carotenoids protect plants from ultraviolet damage. In humans carotenoids are supposed to reflect light rays and convert light energy to chemical energy, as they do in plants.

They also reduce the damaging activity of free radicals, counteract the immunosuppressive effects of ultraviolet radiation and "scatter" some of the ultraviolet light. Ultraviolet exposure depletes skin beta-carotene levels, making the skin more prone to photodamage.

In a German study (*Eur. J. Derm.*, 1996: 200-5), women were given a daily dose of 30 mg. of beta-carotene for two months before exposure to the sun. After two weeks' controlled exposure, they had an increase over controls in their numbers of Lagerhans cells, an important component of the skin's immune system, which is markedly diminished by the sun's radiation. *What Doctors Don't Tell You* columnist Harald Gaier routinely advises everyone over 9 years old to take a daily supplement of 7500 IU vita-

min A, starting with the night before the first exposure, until their skin is used to the sun.

Vitamin E and other antioxidants (selenium, vitamin C) are useful to ward off the damaging effects of
ultraviolet light.

Useful Contacts

American Biologics
Mexico S.A. Medical Center
15 Azucenas Street
Tijuana, B.C.
Mexico
1-800-227-4458 or
1-619-429-8200
www.americanbiologics.com

American Holistic Medical Association
6728 Old McLean Village Drive
McLean, VA 22101
1-703-556-9728
(Referral list - $10)
www.holisticmedicine.org (Free referral list)

American International Hospital and Clinic
(5 branch locations)
3455 Salt Creek Lane, Suite 2000
Arlington Heights, IL 60005
1-800-FOR-HELP
www.cancercenter.com

American Natural Hygiene Society
PO Box 30630
Tampa, FL 33630
1-813-855-6607
www.anhs.org

Ralph Moss
Equinox Press
144 St John's Place,
Brooklyn, NY 11217
718-636 4433 or 636 1679
Provides the same services as People Against Cancer.

Further Reading

Michael Lerner. *Choices in Healing: Integrating the Best of Conventional and Complementary Approaches to Cancer* (MIT Press, 1994).

Ralph W Moss. *Questioning Chemotherapy* (Equinox Press, 1995). (Equinox Press: 144 St John's Place, Brooklyn, NY 11217).

Ralph W Moss. *Cancer Therapy. The Independent Consumer's Guide to Non-Toxic Treatment and Prevention* (Equinox Press, 1995).

Ralph W Moss. *The Cancer Industry* (Equinox Press, 1996).

Ross Pelton and Lee Overholser. *Alternatives in Cancer Therapy: The Complete Guide to Non-traditional Treatments* (Fireside, 1994).

Richard A Passwater. *Cancer Prevention and Nutritional Therapies* (Keats Publishing, 1978).

Sandra Goodman. *Nutrition and Cancer: State of the Art* (Green Library Publications, 1995). (Green Library: 9 Rickett Street, London SW6 1RU).

Liz Hodgkinson & Jane Metcalfe. *The Bristol Experience* (Vermilion, 1995).

Richard Evans. *Making the Right Choice: Treatment Options in Cancer Surgery* (Avery, 1995).

Hulda Regehr Clark. *The Cure for All Cancers* (ProMotion Publishing, 1993).

Dr Gerald B Dermer. *The Immortal Cell: Why Cancer Research Fails* (Avery, 1994).

Vernon Coleman. *Power over Cancer* (European Medical Journal, 1996).

Aveline Kushi. *The Macrobiotic Cancer Prevention Cookbook* (Avery 1988).

Jan Dries. *The Dries Cancer Diet* (Element Books, 1997).

Books by

Vital Health Publishing

Lecithin and Health, Frank Orthoefer, Ph.D.

Natural Body Basics: Making Your Own Cosmetics, Dorie Byers, R.N.

Anoint Yourself with Oil for Radiant Health, David Richard

My Whole Food ABC's, David Richard and Susan Cavaciuti

Taste Life! The Organic Choice, ed. David Richard and Dorie Byers, R.N.

Stevia Rebaudiana: Nature's Sweet Secret, David Richard

Stevia Sweet Recipes: Sugar-Free – Naturally!, Jeffrey Goettemoeller

Recetas Dulces con Stevia: Sin-Azucar – Naturalmente!, Jeffrey Goettemoeller

Wheatgrass: Superfood for a New Millennium, Li Smith

Nutrition in a Nutshell: Build Health and Slow Down the Aging Process, Bonnie C. Minsky, M.A.

Energy for Life: How to Manage Your Metabolic Potential, George Redmon, Ph.D., N.D.

Taste Life: The Organic Recipe Book, ed. Leslie Cerier

Enhancement Books

The Healer: Heart and Hearth, John Diamond, M.D.

The Healing Power of Blake: A Distillation, ed. John Diamond, M.D.

The Way of the Pulse: Drumming with Spirit, John Diamond, M.D.

The Veneration of Life: Through the Disease to the Soul, John Diamond, M.D.

Life Enhancement Through Music, John Diamond, M.D.

Facets of Diamond: Aspects of a Healer, John Diamond, M.D.

Vital Health Publishing/Enhancement Books

P.O. Box 544
Bloomingdale, IL 60108
630-876-0426
www.vitalhealth.net
vitalhealth@compuserve.com